Review of *A Fresh Wellness Mindset: Personalize Y*
about Gluten by Tam John, BA, NTP:

A Fresh Wellness Mindset is a refreshing and needed addition to the myriad of books written on the subject of nutrition and wellness. So many authors of nutrition take the position that they have discovered the one way and that their way is the only way. There never has been, nor will there ever be, one way for everyone because everyone is different and the one perfect diet for one person (the author of the book perhaps) is not necessarily the answer for everyone else. What is the perfect diet for them could easily make you sick!

Tam John's book is, on the other hand, a guide to self discovery that will lead her readers to the diet that works for them. No more "diet of the month" approaches here. Tam carefully explains the nuances of important topics like gluten intolerance and grain consumption. For some individuals grains are a horrible food, but for others, they can be a useful and enjoyable part of a healthy diet. She has made the journey herself from poor health back to vitality and now is compelled to help others on their journey!

A Fresh Wellness Mindset is a well referenced and scientifically accurate guide that can be used by an individual on their own journey or in conjunction with a Wellness Practitioner. Well done!

Gray L. Graham, BA, NTP

Founder of the Nutritional Therapy Association, Inc.

Author of *Pottenger's Prophecy, How Food Can Reset Genes for Wellness or Illness*

A
FRESH
WELLNESS
MINDSET

Personalize Your Food Life
&
Find Your Truth about Gluten

By Tam John, BA, NTP

© Copyright 2018
ISBN-13: 978-1981340323
Library of Congress Control Number: 2017919209
CreateSpace Independent Publishing Platform, North Charleston, SC

Because of the dynamic nature of the internet, any web addresses/URLs or links contained in this book may have changed since publication. Therefore they may no longer be valid.

The views expressed in this book are solely those of the author.

This book is not a substitute for qualified medical care. It is not intended to replace the advice of a qualified health professional, treat, diagnose, cure or prevent disease. If you know or suspect that you have a health problem, you should consult with a qualified health professional.

The author specifically disclaims any responsibility, liability, loss, or damage caused or alleged to be caused, or risk, personal or otherwise, that is incurred as a consequence, directly or indirectly of the use, application or interpretation of any information presented in this book. The author is not a licensed practitioner, physician, or medical professional and offers no medical diagnoses or treatments.

This book is for informational purposes. This book has not been reviewed by the U.S. Food and Drug Administration (FDA). Always consult with your primary care Physician or Naturopathic Doctor before beginning or modifying any diet, exercise, or lifestyle program, and physicians should be informed of all nutritional changes.

www.TamJohn.com

Dedication

For Daisy, my best girl

Love You Pea

Table of Contents

Preface

Dear Reader,

In what I perceived as 'all of a sudden', signs and symptoms rearing their ugliness told me something was way off as to how my body was functioning. I struggled to understand what was happening and what to do to reverse it. Although I wanted to blame aging, I was only in my early forties. I knew this was not normal aging.

Up to this time of my life, I glided into each new day with exuberance. I viewed life as an adventure. Now my energy lagged way behind my standards. My body was rampant with painful sensations; sore joints and muscles; severe digestive distress and an overall sense of foreboding heaviness. Regularly I had huge headaches lasting for days that sent me to bed. Once the pain subsided, I was left with feeling an imprint in my head of where the headache had been. Life as I knew it was gone.

Rather than running my business and household with enthusiasm leftover for exploring the great Colorado outdoors, I felt zapped. Up to then, seven mile hikes, a full morning of snow shoeing, 10 or 15 miles of mountain biking, being on a competitive tennis team or taking a spur of the moment vacation to a city or country I had never visited were routinely part of my life. Now I was relegated to down shifting; going to work and home and nothing much more. Rather than a busy schedule in and out of the office, visiting clients around the Denver metropolitan area, I sought to be stationed in my office the vast majority of time. Seriously concerned, I felt like I was spiraling and questioned if my life was sustainable.

My Physician ran tests which came back in the normal range and they assured me I was fine. I soon sought the help of a Naturopath because I continued to feel worse. I engaged with this natural practitioner for hormone testing via a saliva panel and a detailed intake interview. The supplement regimen they recommended resulted in feeling worse with more outwardly visible discomfort revealing inflammation.

I made a trail to practitioner after practitioner. I engaged with bio-feedback, Reiki, Acupuncture, energy healing, chelation, Iridology, Functional Chiropractors, and other Doctors. I sought answers to the questions: What was going on with my body and how could I fix it? While I found value in all of these modalities to one extent or another, none of them clicked as a means for restoration of me.

The information I received from practitioners about food as a source for wellness was limited and inconsistent. Deeply I believed it made sense that food should be able to nourish me to health, but I began to doubt my choices. Up to this time, I thought I had a pretty clean diet and made healthy choices. I knew I wasn't perfect, but according to my Physician's input along with the standards and guidelines I knew, I ate pretty well. I didn't have an obvious reaction to anything I ate.

What I came to learn is that it is imperative to know what choices are healthy for us before we can make healthy choices. Everybody is beautifully bio-individual with unique bio-chemistry. Our bodies deal with input of food, drink and lifestyle differently even though we share similar function. If we aren't digesting food well, even the best of food is detrimental. Overtime the wrong choices of food, drink, and lifestyle (overwork, stress, not enough rest) create a cascade of dysfunction and ultimately breakdown the body.

I found even the so called personalized eating plans to suit body types and other factors like blood type might be a good guide to making healthful choices, but I did not find one plan or model that was an exact fit. In fact, I found a couple of major 'errors' for my body with recommendations based on 'type'.

I have learned the value of listening to my body and how I feel. We all have within our reach the ability to make the best food, drink and lifestyle choices in each moment based on what is available and how our choices make us feel. I got my health and my life back by doing exactly that.

I let go of my corporate career to enter a graduate level holistic nutrition program and earn my certification as a Nutritional Therapy Practitioner (NTP). Now I guide people with a bio-individual approach to help them know which choices are healthy (for them) and how to eat right and live well.

The human body is designed for wellness. When we give it the right input of food, drink and lifestyle it can gracefully fuel us for life with vitality. Amazingly, the body loves simple, delicious and satisfying choices which are healthy for us.

With deep gratitude for my journey back to wellness I am sharing what I have learned personally and professionally. It is one of my greatest life wishes that this book is pivotal for you to live optimally with wellness. because Wellness is True Happiness™.

Be Your Beautiful Self,

Tam John

Introduction

Within the United States there is a trend or even a movement occurring that is leading to a gluten free diet. This Gluten Free Movement (GFM) is necessary in some cases where the intake of gluten is causing health issues. In other cases there are personal choices being made that may or may not be beneficial to the individual. A significant focus of this book is to help the reader understand when a gluten free diet is beneficial and when some alternative other than going entirely gluten free forever may actually be a healthier alternative.

Many people have serious health reasons not to eat gluten containing grains. This group includes those Celiac diagnosed or Non-Celiac Gluten Sensitive (NCGS) persons. The numbers of people who must avoid gluten for the sake of their health are increasing by leaps and bounds. Rightly, people wonder what is happening with so many of us being sickened by the food we eat.

Other people avoid gluten because they have heard and believe it must be bad, given the pop culture, how they think it makes them feel, and hearing the distressing experiences of those with Celiac or NCGS. They wonder if a myriad of symptoms including digestive discomfort, unwanted weight, aches, pains, mood and other discomfort is due to ingestion of gluten. They think they might feel better without gluten, but aren't entirely sure. In many cases they are not at all consistent in the avoidance of gluten.

Some avoid gluten when they choose to and/or when it is convenient to make a gluten free selection. Consuming gluten may precipitate feelings of guilt and/or may actually lead to the escalation of unwanted symptoms when they don't avoid gluten. This escalation of symptoms reinforces the belief that consuming gluten is the culprit.

People are rightfully confused with the trending information concerning gluten. Uncertain about their choice to consume or avoid gluten, uncomfortable symptoms remain part of their experience. Much of the ugly information about modern (processed and refined) gluten is accurate. However, much of the information about gluten is inaccurate or not 'bio-individually' accurate in all cases when considering gluten containing products as an entire category of food, and when consumed as nature intended.

People with contemporary lives need accurate information about how to make food choices to serve up nutrition as fuel for their bodies for energy, growth, restoration and repair. This book will explore the seriousness of the ramifications of ingesting the 'modern' highly processed and refined forms of gluten.

It serves as a resource guide to understand gluten and the health ramifications for those whose bodies are irritated by gluten ingestion. This book is a resource guide to give people step by step guidance to eliminate gluten and possibly restore bodily function so they can eat 'good' gluten without issue.

This book is for everyone, whether they avoid or consume gluten. It is resource for transforming a Standard American Diet (SAD) into a personalized yummy nutrient dense real food diet healthy for you, Dear Reader.

You can't make healthy choices until you know which choices are healthy for you. All 'healthy' food isn't healthy for everyone. Learning which choices are healthy for you gives you a means to choose wisely. Personalized food choices which agree with you need not break your resources of time or budget.

This book is written to help everyone unravel their own personal wellness puzzle and is a guide to personalize food choices for life. You will learn how to read your body; how to make healthful choices; and how to love food that loves you back. When you learn to choose food optimal for your body you won't need to diet again. Without dieting you can feel a sense of deep satisfaction with your food without the deprivation diets imply.

The happy result gives you a solid foundation of optimal wellness to establish better feeling energy and vitality today, tonight and for life. Personalized food choices fit your fingerprint perfectly.

This book will show you how to implement sustainable routines without boredom and just the right amount of effort for your life. This book will show you how to erase confusion and find your personal truth about gluten. It will support you to reset digestion and blood sugar regulation by developing habits for making great choices of food you love.

Reading this book, you will get lots of reliable information, resources, tips and ideas. You deserve to feel your best, abundant with energy and wellness to live your life fully.

Let's Get Started!

This book is not a substitute for qualified medical care. It is not intended to replace the advice of a qualified health professional, treat, diagnose, cure or prevent disease. If you know or suspect that you have a health problem, you should consult with a qualified health professional.

The author specifically disclaims any responsibility, liability, loss, or damage caused or alleged to be caused, or risk, personal or otherwise, that is incurred as a consequence, directly or indirectly of the use, application or interpretation of any information presented in this book. The author is not a licensed practitioner, physician, or medical professional and offers no medical diagnoses or treatments.

This book is for informational purposes. This book has not been reviewed by the U.S. Food and Drug Administration (FDA). Always consult with your primary care Physician or Naturopathic Doctor before beginning or modifying any diet, exercise, or lifestyle program, and physicians should be informed of all nutritional changes.

Chapter 1

A Brief History:
Human Consumption of Gluten Containing Grains

"Everywhere the grain stood ripe and the hot afternoon was full of the smell of the ripe wheat, like the smell of bread baking in an oven. The breath of the wheat and the sweet clover passed him like pleasant things in a dream."

~Willa Cather, *O Pioneers*!

Humans have been eating wheat and other gluten containing grains for around 30,000 years. There is archaeological evidence of flour from wild cereal grains made in (what is now) Europe from around 30,000 years ago. (Douillard, 2017) Wheat began being cultivated as a crop around 10,000 years ago. The cultivation of wheat as a crop helped create more reliable and accessible sources of food, allowing humans to move from being hunters and gathers to living in a more stable, agricultural society. (Murray, 2014)

Since wheat and other gluten containing grains have been part of the human diet for tens of thousands of years, we wonder why the consumption of wheat in recent years has become a detrimental health issue for so many people. Many of us used to eat wheat and gluten containing grains without issue. Many of us remember being coaxed or outright told by our Moms and Grandmothers to choose the wheat bread because it was a healthy staple of life. Some people report when they travel to Europe they don't have an issue eating wheat and other gluten containing bread, and other food. Wheat remains a staple of life for many people on this planet. We wonder why this huge issue, more like a movement, has swept across America.

Roughly two million Americans diagnosed Celiac and those with NCGS should not eat wheat or other gluten containing grains. Many would argue no one should eat gluten, ever.

These opponents to ever eating any gluten say it isn't a matter of not tolerating gluten... Everyone is intolerant of gluten because they say gluten is toxic. Emphasis is on *how* the body is expressing intolerance of gluten, not *if* the body is expressing intolerance of gluten.

As a society we may be drawn to the idea of making one food or one thing out to be all bad when an issue is complex with many layers and intricacies. We resolve something must take the blame. The more concise the answer is, the more acceptable it is for a society to come together on the matter. In other eras in recent history, the enemy has been cholesterol, anything with fat, and carbohydrates. These health concepts once thought of as 'truth' have now been set aside as untruth. For some time now, gluten is deemed an enemy of the body by many if not most.

With impartiality let us peel back the intricate layers of what has become a problematic food for many. To consider gluten's viability as friend or foe to the body consider how wheat has changed from being consumed as a whole food to being consumed as an overly processed and refined food ingredient. Today's modern and highly processed and refined wheat is barely recognizable from the time wheat berries were gathered and eaten by nomadic cultures. True stone milling and grinding is a thing of the past for the vast majority.

Wheat is one of the most cultivated crops in the United States. Seldom is a wheat berry found for consumption. Instead, wheat cultivation in the US is subsidized by the government and grown for mass production with pesticides, fertilizer and other chemicals. Wheat is mass harvested, stored, milled and refined into processed food products combined with artificial ingredients and usually a lot of sugar or sugary derivatives. Government subsidized commodity crops such as wheat are cheap, making it very attractive to food manufacturers, hence its dominance on manufactured and processed food labels. Mass production creates need for mass storage which makes the crop susceptible to molds and fungi. Synthetic vitamins and minerals are often added back to the finished food product. The over processing of wheat applies to other gluten containing grains as well. Nourishment is severely diminished with all the processing and mass storage of the grain.

While wheat and gluten containing grains as food have changed significantly over the course of millennia, the human body has not changed all that much in those same years. New versions of food with wheat dominant ingredients are much different than nature intended. Adulterated foods fuss with proper bodily function. Energy creation, digestion, immunity, blood sugar regulation, elimination, detoxification, reproduction, strength and structure of the human body object to the new versions of wheat and other gluten containing grains. When bodily function 'objects' to food it is a reflection of the burden the food is placing on your brilliantly interconnected body. The objection is expressed as signs and symptoms telling you your body is in distress and asking for support. Something isn't working well. We weren't designed to absorb and assimilate new fangled food altered from its original form.

Gluten in its modern form has become bad news and seems to be getting worse as grocery store shelves are proliferated with heavily processed foods with wheat leading the ingredient list. Avoiding food products with modern gluten grains leading a long ingredient list on the labels of laboratory made food is a vote for change in what shows up on store shelves. As a plus this gives your body a reprieve from adulterated food. Big grocery will only change in response to how we choose to spend our grocery dollars. When we stop buying anything, the producer will stop making it.

Some people may choose to be done with gluten forever, even if they are not Celiac. They've gotten sick and experienced awful feelings of distress and discomfort from a food supply gone wrong. They may have seen others suffer and think it safest to avoid gluten containing grains as much as they can if not altogether. They accept the notion of all gluten being poisonous. Bestselling books written about the damaging and detrimental effects of gluten containing grains with wheat as a target, including the blame for too much weight around the mid body as wheat's fault, resonate as their truth.

The connection purported to eating modern wheat and too much weight around the body's middle section is easy to make. Processed wheat quickly turns to glucose in the body. Excess glucose is stored as fat and triglycerides. It makes sense wheat would take credit for too much middle body fat. Too much middle body fat reflects excess wheat (gluten) containing processed foods, too much sugar and other food (often starches) quickly turning to glucose in the body. Simply giving up wheat (and other gluten containing grains) and continuing to eat many other foods that quickly convert to glucose will result in the same issue of too much middle body weight or whatever your body's expression (signs and symptoms) is.

Continuing behavior of eating problematic and symptomatic foods may likely pronounce current issues and degrade future wellness status. Recurring signs and symptoms are not normal. Too often people under consider and ignore persistent tummy troubles or skin breakouts or rashes or whatever manifests outwardly as distress from their internal terrain. When you diet or give up wheat containing foods for a period you may feel and look better for a while. When you revert to the behavior which got you where you did not want to be you fall back to where you were and sometimes farther back. Restoration has not been complete and/or you've reintroduced the same quality of food which creates the problem.

Part-time gluten avoidance for gluten intolerance or Celiac disease, or a diet to meet a goal like weight loss or a big event can be a vicious cycle. With a Celiac this behavior is very destructive and must be avoided to avoid more internal destruction. Humans explain the bad feelings, signs and symptoms away as aging, genetic ('my Grandpa had that') as if it is a life sentence. We tell ourselves we've always had a weight problem, anxiety runs in the family, or some other explanation to which we remain perplexed and uncomfortable. Vicious cycles are vicious. They create more stress when you need relief. You deserve to permanently feel better.

Even if you suspect gluten is an issue for you although you haven't been diagnosed Celiac, avoiding gluten grains is a reasonable step to allow your body to restore from the destruction gluten can cause which causes discomforting symptoms. Those symptoms (discussed in detail in Chapter 2) are the body's message that something is amiss and a food may be the culprit linked to distress.

If you must avoid gluten there has never been a better time to be gluten free. Although it can seem overwhelming to remove a food so dominant in your pantry and eating regimen, foods free of gluten are abundantly available to satisfy, energize and nourish you. This book will show you how to make choices naturally nourishing for your body that are entirely free of gluten. You can experience restoration and resolve from the distress gluten can play in your body once you give your body the right food.

Beyond learning how easy and satisfying it can be to eat a food free of gluten, you will learn to make choices your body will thrive on. Thriving means your digestion and uptake of nutrients will be ideal. Optimal digestion plays into stable blood sugar regulation. These two functions are the basis for everything else working well in the body including energy creation, detoxification, rejuvenation, restoration and growth. It is inevitable you will naturally feel better when your body is well functioning.

The next chapter will pinpoint Celiac disease, its signs/symptoms and possible links to gluten intolerance be it Celiac or Non-Celiac Gluten Sensitivity or some intolerance approaching either condition.

Chapter 2

The Beginning of a Gluten Free Movement (GFM)

"History is the sum total of the things
that could have been avoided."

~Konrad Adenauer

Before the mass production of gluten with artificial means, and before chemical components dominated the growing and over processing of wheat as an agricultural crop, there has been evidence of Celiac disease. This indicates some people's bio-chemistry is not aligned with the healthful consumption of wheat or gluten grains.

Celiac disease was observed as early as the second century although its cause wasn't identified until the 20th century (http://www.csac-eliacs.org/history_of_celiac_disease.jsp). Celiac disease was referred to as Non Tropical Sprue Disease when identified in adults. The disease is commonly seen as failure to thrive or malabsorption of nutrients resulting in malnutrition. Today the common difference between having Celiac disease or Non Celiac Gluten Sensitivity (NCGS) has to do with the HLA gene which provides instructions for making a protein critical for the immune system (https://ghr.nlm.nih.gov/gene/HLA-B).

In 250 A.D., Aretaeus of Cappadocia included detailed descriptions of an unnamed disease in his writings. When describing his patients he referred to them as "koiliakos," which meant "suffering in the bowels." Francis Adams translated these observations from Greek to English for the Sydenham Society of England in 1856. He thus gave sufferers the moniker "celiacs" or "coeliacs." Thus Europe uses the spelling coeliac disease with the "o". (http://www.csaceliacs.org/-history_of_celiac_disease.jsp)

In the late 1800s Samuel Gee, MD, working with children and adults with Celiac Disease in the UK stated, "To regulate the food is the main part of treatment. The allowance of farinaceous foods must be small, but if the patient can be cured at all, it must be by means of diet." (http://www.csaceliacs.org/history_of_celiac_-disease.jsp) Farinaceous foods are those made with flour, wheat or similar meal and contain starch such as bread.

In 1952, Willem Karel Dicke, MD linked wheat proteins to the cause of Celiac Disease and described the histological damage to the intestinal mucosa.

According to the Celiac Support Association ®, **in 1986** the evidence of Celiac Disease was said to be 1 in 5000 and a 1 in 10 incidence with close relative. (http://www.csaceliacs.org/history_of_celiac_disease.jsp)

Dr. Anne Ferguson, **in 1998** at the University of Edinburgh, noted the wide spectrum of antigen-induced mucosal changes with gluten-sensitivity beyond the strict definition of celiac disease. (http://onlinelibrary.wiley.com/doi/10.1046/j.13652796.1996.41875000.x/full)

According to University of Chicago Celiac Disease Center the prevalence of Celiac Disease at the time of this writing in 2017 is 1 in 133. (http://www.uchospitals.edu/pdf/uch_00-7937.pdf)

Celiac Disease Defined

You have to be eating gluten to develop Celiac disease….. None of us digest gluten completely since it is a large, complex protein that remains mainly resistant to our normal intestinal enzymes. (Green, 2016) Some of us express gluten intolerance more than others whether it manifests as Celiac disease, NCGS, or our body just doesn't digest it so well leaving us more or fewer signs and symptoms.

Celiac disease is a multisystem autoimmune disorder whose main target of injury is the small intestine. (Green, 2016) The small intestine is where more than 90% of nutrient absorption occurs. When digestion isn't working well and undigested food passes from the stomach to the small intestine, nutrient absorption suffers. The delicate epithelial lining of the small intestine becomes damaged from undigested food (like gluten grains). The body perceives the undigested food (like gluten) as a foreign invader. This is the beginning of auto-immunity. Individual diversity at a bio-chemical level explains the accompanying vast array of symptoms and signs reflecting the presentation of Celiac disease and gluten sensitivity.

The body needs both inflammation and anti-inflammation to moderate healthy body function. When the body determines a foreign invader is present, inflammation increases and is out of balance with anti-inflammation. Undigested gluten passing through and between mucosal cells lining the intestinal tract further compromises healthy function. Burden of stress in the body reflects outwardly as the signs and symptoms of dysfunction. Excess inflammation destroys healthy tissue. The small intestine is lined with villi which are very thin but finger like projections which filter the passing of nutrients from the small intestine to the blood stream. Villi become damaged so nutrients are no longer able to pass through for absorption. The vicious cycle progresses as the immune system makes more antibodies to food proteins like gluten grains. More food sensitivities may develop. The body becomes fatigued. Symptoms, although they may be similar, arc bio-individual to each person and present outwardly reflecting damage and nutrient deficiencies.

Much of the damage caused by Celiac disease occurs where you can't see or sometimes even feel it – within your digestive system. (Murray, 2014) Once symptoms are present, destruction of healthy function in the body has progressed. Sometimes the body's reaction to gluten occurs over time and in others it is fast and traumatic.

Murray (2014) describes the following terms Doctors may use when talking about Celiac disease, to describe different types of the disease. They include **Classical Celiac disease**. This is used when the main symptoms are indications of (nutrient) malabsorption. Instead of inclusion of malabsorption, **Nonclassical Celiac disease** reflects abdominal pain, constipation, fatigue or anemia. **Asymptomatic Celiac disease** is silent Celiac disease. These patients are diagnosed through screening programs because they are deemed to be at high risk, due to close relatives with Celiac disease. **Potential Celiac disease** is sometimes referred to as latent celiac disease. These are people without symptoms who are considered high risk for the future development of the disease. Their small intestine lining looks normal but blood tests are positive for Celiac disease. **Subclinical Celiac disease** is used to refer to mild or seemingly unrelated signs and symptoms that aren't normally associated with Celiac disease, but raise suspicion the individual may have Celiac disease.

Signs/Symptoms of Gluten Issues

Celiac disease, gluten sensitivity and intolerance uniquely affect each person. The variance of signs and symptoms is a reflection of the unique bio-chemistry of each person. Each person's body reacts to stressors differently. Symptoms commonly occur in the digestive system because the issue is based on maldigestion of the proteins in gluten. One person might have diarrhea and abdominal pain, while another person may be irritable or depressed (think Gut-Brain Axis). Irritability is one of the most common symptoms in children. Some people have no symptoms. (https://vsearch.nlm.nih.gov/vivisimo/cgi-bin/query-meta?v%3Aproject=medlineplus&v%3Asources=medline-plus-bundle&query=celiac+disease&_ga=1.243545543.33137172-4.1487373416)

According to Mayo Clinic (http://www.mayoclinic.org/diseases-conditions/celiac-disease/symptoms-causes/dxc-20214627), the signs and symptoms of Celiac disease can vary greatly and are different in children and adults. The most common signs for adults are diarrhea, fatigue and weight loss. Adults may also experience bloating and gas, abdominal pain, nausea, constipation, and vomiting.

However, more than half of adults with Celiac disease have signs and symptoms that are not related to the digestive system, including:

❖ Anemia, usually resulting from iron deficiency
❖ Loss of bone density (osteoporosis) or softening of bone (osteomalacia)
❖ Itchy, blistery skin rash (dermatitis herpetiformis)
❖ Damage to dental enamel
❖ Mouth ulcers
❖ Headaches and fatigue
❖ Nervous system injury, including numbness and tingling in the feet and hands, possible problems with balance, and cognitive impairment
❖ Joint pain
❖ Reduced functioning of the spleen (hyposplenism)
❖ Acid reflux and heartburn

In children under 2 years old, typical signs and symptoms of Celiac disease include:

❖ Vomiting
❖ Chronic diarrhea
❖ Swollen belly
❖ Failure to thrive
❖ Poor appetite
❖ Muscle wasting

Older children may experience:

❖ Diarrhea
❖ Constipation
❖ Weight loss
❖ Irritability

❖ Short stature

❖ Delayed puberty

❖ Neurological symptoms, including attention-deficit/hyper-activity disorder (ADHD), learning disabilities, headaches, lack of muscle coordination and seizures

Mayo Clinic goes on to say, Dermatitis herpetiformis is an itchy, blistering skin disease that stems from intestinal gluten intolerance. The rash usually occurs on the elbows, knees, torso, scalp and buttocks. It is often associated with changes to the lining of the small intestine identical to those of celiac disease, but the disease may not produce noticeable digestive symptoms.

While Gastrointestinal (GI) symptoms like diarrhea have traditionally been associated with Celiac disease, Doctors now see symptoms reflecting malabsorption to be common.

According to Murray (2014), signs and symptoms of Celiac disease may be… Cognitive and memory problems, balance problems, hair loss, lung changes, heart problems, anemia, infertility, bone changes, joint pain, numbness, tingling, swelling, headaches and fatigue, night vision problems, nosebleeds, mouth ulcers, esophageal changes, shrunken spleen, stomach problems, GI problems, cancer, bruising, itchy skin rash.

A Physician can advise on a variety of labs and diagnostic tests to confirm Celiac disease. This is important when destructive and depleting signs & symptoms are present. If Celiac disease is not the cause, further examination with a Physician can find the source of the signs and symptoms. It is important to get to the bottom of what is ailing you to intervene if disease is manifesting. Murray (2014) also says, other conditions like IBS (Irritable Bowel Syndrome), chronic fatigue syndrome, fibromyalgia or unexplained nerve inflammation (idiopathic neuropathy) may mask an underlying gluten problem if Celiac disease isn't ruled out.

Reasons beyond a Celiac diagnosis or being NCGS, to withdraw gluten containing food and products may include:

❖ What seems like obvious sensitivity to gluten containing food and products with signs & symptoms a Celiac or NCGS person experiences

❖ Concern about how gluten containing grains are grown and or processed for consumption

❖ Theories about gluten consumption contributing to obesity, abdominal fat or depression feel like they may fit your wellness scenario

Going gluten free for a short period of time (or moorkishorly) in unlikely to bring sustained improvement of function or lessening of symptoms. Complete consistent removal of gluten from the diet is necessary for those with a Celiac diagnosis and those who are NCGS.

For others who wish to know if gluten ingestion may be at the core of their symptoms, complete and consistent removal of gluten may have positive impact toward sign/symptom reduction and support restoration of function. Entire removal of gluten and supporting functional restoration with food and supplements with the guidance of a Physician or qualified practitioner can be health supportive. Gradual reintroduction of gluten grains after restoration may be viable for some who are not diagnosed Celiac. Chapter 9 details more about food intolerances and allergies, restoration and possible reintroduction.

Possible Links to Gluten Intolerance

Auto-immunity (AI): AI occurs when the body's immune system attacks its own healthy cells and tissues. According to University of Chicago Celiac Disease Center, Celiac Disease is an inherited auto-immune disorder that affects the digestive process of the small intestine. (http://www.uchospitals.edu/pdf/uch_007937.pdf)

According to Johns Hopkins Medicine, 'Clinical and epidemiologic evidence as well as data from experimental animals demonstrate that a tendency to develop autoimmune disease is inherited. This tendency may be large or small depending on the disease but, in general, close relatives are more likely to develop the same or a related autoimmune disease. A number of genes have been implicated in causing autoimmune disease, primarily genes related to the human major histocompatibility complex called HLA.' (http://autoimmune.pathology.jhmi.edu/faqs.cfm) These genes provide instructions for making proteins that help the immune system distinguish the body's own proteins from foreign proteins produced by pathogens or found in foods. The vast majority of people with Celiac disease have either the HLA-DQ2 gene or the HLA-DQ8 gene; although, there are also many people who have these genes but do not have Celiac disease. This means that having these genes is typically necessary but not sufficient to cause sensitivity to gluten. In addition to these genes, a number of other genes have been associated with Celiac diseases, although they do not seem to have as much influence on whether or not you will develop the disease. (https://www.khanacademy.org/test-prep/nclex-rn/gastrointestinal-diseases/celiac-disease-rn/a/what-is-celiac-disease)

Genetic: According to Green (2016), there is a definite genetic influence that is demonstrated by the prevalence of Celiac disease in families and in identical twins, but not all the genes have been conclusively identified.

Lifestyle: Altering genetic expression with the food you eat, along with lifestyle choices, and environment (stress, sleep, etc.) may be important to overall wellness as demonstrated by the exciting developments with epigenetics.   Modifying mainstream lifestyle factors including what you eat and drink; how food is grown, preserved & prepared; how you treat illness; the extensive use of antibiotics and other drugs that alter digestion and damage intestinal lining; and over the counter medications that also impact the digestive system will likely impact sensitivity to gluten.   Imagine altering/improving a genetic predisposition by simply choosing real food personally appealing.   Eating in a calm state can have a big positive impact on digestive function, as described in Chapter 7.   Wellness results from healthy input of food that is right for your body and lifestyle choices.

The impact of stress cannot be overlooked as a contributor to dis-ease.   Stress may seem endless in busy modern lives unless you make choices to fortify wellness and optimal function by lightening your stress load.   Just because 'everyone' is stressed does not make the symptoms of stress normal for the body or any less detrimental.   For optimal wellness, you must find reprieve from overwhelming stress to relieve your body and mind.

Modern lives are jammed with busy schedules and factors sometimes seemingly out of control.   The human body's management of cortisol (a stress hormone) is meant to be primarily released by the adrenal glands at the perception of stress.   Cortisol is highly effective in preparing the body to react to stress (like a charging tiger in the days of ancestral man).   It also gets involved in digestive function and blood sugar regulation to a greater or lesser extent, depending on the strength of those functions independent of cortisol's assistance.   And since the body perceives the need to release cortisol in a life- saving activity (like running from a charging tiger) the same as getting caught at a stop light when you are late, the release of cortisol for stress reasons is epidemic.

Optimizing digestion and blood sugar regulation supports cortisol release as relegated to its stress fighting role.   Diminishing stress and the body's perception of stress will be all the more favorable for healthy cortisol regulation.   Even though cortisol is very effective as Mother Nature designed it, primarily for the stress response, its release is catabolic – it breaks down the body.   Too frequent cortisol release and its dysregulation can become 'catastrophic' for healthy function.

The global reach of media giving rampant bad news reports, as well as our devices giving us more information than we can possibly process, contributes to cortisol dysregulation. News reports and electromagnetic frequency (EMF) emissions from our devices are two more inputs which drive up cortisol dysregulation. Do yourself a healthy service by dialing back stressful modern-day inputs.

Sometimes the sudden onset of Celiac or NCGS and its symptoms are thought to be the result of a 'Stress Trigger'. According to Murray (2014), sometimes for reasons that aren't clear, Celiac disease emerges after some form of trauma, such as an infection, physical injury, the stress of pregnancy, severe stress or surgery. Stress and trauma incurred as a child and adult alters function. (http://acestudy.org/the-ace-score.html)

It is never too late to begin de-stressing for better functional health. Here are some ideas to de-stress:

❖ Seek out activities to increase your motion at a comfortable pace. Your body is designed for movement.
❖ Get out of doors for 'outdoor therapy'. Being in nature is restorative.
❖ Simply sit with a great book without distraction.
❖ Find 10 minutes for quiet contemplation once or twice every day.
❖ Turn off the TV and put on relaxing music.
❖ Turn off devices an hour or more before bed.
❖ Don't keep your devices on the bedside table.
❖ Say no when you want to. Healthy boundaries equate to excellent self-care.

Glyphosate: A compelling peer-reviewed report from two US scientists, proposes that 'glyphosate, the active ingredient in the herbicide, Roundup®, is the most important causal factor of this epidemic [of Celiac disease]. Fish exposed to glyphosate develop digestive problems that are reminiscent of Celiac disease. Celiac disease is associated with imbalances of gut bacteria that can be fully explained by the known effects of glyphosate on gut bacteria. Characteristics of Celiac disease point to impairment in many cytochrome P450 enzymes, which are involved with detoxifying environmental toxins, …' (Samuel & Seneff, 2013)

According to Douillard (2017), the vast majority of the public does not know that in the past 15 years, it is a practice for wheat farmers in certain areas (primarily North and South Dakota and parts of Canada) to spray their wheat fields with Roundup® or glyphosate several days before harvest. Douillard (2017) goes on to say that some experts are linking not only the epidemic of non-celiac gluten sensitivity to ingesting glyphosate, but also the dramatic increase in Celiac disease. Exposure to glyphosate is insidious, as it causes a slow, steady, gradual alteration of the gut microbiome and inflammation of the intestinal tract.

Modern technology using the proliferation of manmade and toxic chemicals in the food supply creates an issue for the body. The human body isn't designed to ingest manmade chemicals. Chemicals also interfere with natural detoxification the body is designed for. According to Green (2016), genetic modification of wheat cannot explain the rise in gluten-related disorders and Celiac disease.

Considering the long history of Celiac disease and NCGS, it makes sense chemicals used for modern crop growing regimes may not be entirely the cause of gluten intolerance. Each body is a brilliant interconnected masterpiece that deals with offenders in similar yet unique ways. Getting to the source of the problem is likely multi-faceted and will remain bio-individually unique for each person. Use common sense when choosing your food and be keenly aware of the possibilities for modern food practices to be disruptive to the body. Modern commercial practices which include chemicals have been intended to feed masses of population not involved in food growth or production, as the world economy and population continues to grow.

When possible, choose foods organically and naturally grown and raised, as nature intended. Your purchases are a vote for what you want to see on store shelves. Marketers and producers deliver more of what sells. Take a positive approach to vote with your choices. Invest your food and dining budget in what you want to see more of.

Microbiome: The microbiome is healthy gut bacteria. Experts don't completely agree on the ideal ratio of microbiome to human cells. Estimates of the ideal ratio vary from 1:1 to 10:1 microbiome to human cells. Microbiome supports the Gut-Brain Axis which plays heavily in healthy digestion and immunity, as well as mood and lessening anxiety and depression.

Brogan (2016) states that glyphosate slaughters beneficial bugs in your intestines, thereby disrupting the balance of your microbiome. When the balance of microbiome is compromised, the digestion of gluten containing grains and other foods would be compromised.

The Gut-Brain Axis and microbiome are largely impacted by lifestyle, birth mode, upbringing from an early age, antibiotics and diet. At least 85% of immunity resides in the gut. When immunity is compromised by the aforementioned factors, the introduction of gluten may create more stress for the immune system and further the likelihood of Celiac disease or NCGS.

Sustained positive real food and drink choices will greatly support microbiome ratios to human cells for optimal function of your digestion and immunity. Fermented and cultured foods like raw cultured veggies and sauerkraut, kombucha, kefir, kvass, miso, tempeh, unsweetened yogurt, sour cream and chutney are some common Gut-Brain Axis friendly foods. A two to four ounce serving daily of these or other fermented foods daily can benefit your microbiome. Introduce fermented foods slowly. Give digestion an opportunity to adjust. Fermented foods are contraindicated for people with histamine issues and very delicate intestinal conditions. Seek the advice of your qualified practitioner or medical professional before making dietary changes.

Digestion – Hippocrates said, "Bad Digestion is the root of all evil." This statement makes good sense when you know digestion is the means by which your body ascertains health status – energy, growth and repair by means of nourishment. Good digestive function is imperative for the assimilation and absorption of nutrients from the food you eat. All the great food in the world is of no benefit without well-functioning digestion. Food must be broken down by digestion to nutrients at the molecular level to generate nourishment and fuel for the trillions of cells in your body.

The body needs real food grown and raised as nature intended because the human body is still grown and raised as nature intended (you know… the birds & bees). Until you are made in a laboratory, neither should your food be made in a laboratory. Combining digestive issues with a modern food supply (overly processed, refined and chemical laden) and lightning fast meals happening simultaneously with the rest of life is detrimental to your best wellness interests.

Whether you grab food from a window and drive away with your hand reaching into the bag for the meal; or you are standing at the kitchen counter wolfing down a bowl of cereal or a frozen laboratory made concoction; or preparing dinner from some open boxes and a microwave; and then sit down with everyone staring at their screens and gulping the food down with a swig of soda – Digestion is compromised by these 'modern' eating scenarios.

Digestion is a parasympathetic process. Parasympathetic processes only happen when we are at rest. You must take your foot off the gas pedal of life to have the benefit of healthy digestion. Digestion begins in the brain where the senses tell us that food is coming. Digestive enzymes begin to be released. Carbohydrate digestion begins in the mouth where salivary amylase is released. Food is broken down by mechanical means with your tongue and chewing. More chewing of carbohydrates means better carbohydrate digestion because it is here, in the mouth, where salivary amylase is released. Four chews and a gulp isn't enough to facilitate proper digestion. You must chew food to become a paste and then liquid before it travels to the stomach. When food enters the stomach wholly intact, you are compromised. It is a set up for dis-ease and a host to a multitude of downstream issues. It is no wonder the body would have an issue digesting gluten proteins and many other foods commonly seen as difficult to digest (like dairy).

Supplementing with digestive enzymes and aids may help the body digest gluten or other proteins and carbohydrates. The body can't replace proper function with a supplement though. Digestive supplements should be used with caution. The epithelial lining is delicate and may be damaged with a too high dosage or the wrong kind of supplementation for your body and issue. Too few supplements won't have a beneficial impact. Don't put anything unhelpful in your body, risk their adversity and waste your resources.

High quality digestive aids may have their place, especially as a bridge, to restore the body's stand-alone function. When choosing digestive supplements, work with a qualified practitioner to test efficacy for your body and be certain you are getting high quality supplements. Without testing, supplementation may be counterproductive. Some supplements contain fillers not on the label and even heavy metals. Caution must be taken to know the product, its ingredients and its manufacturer. Each body may have a 'preference' for one supplement over another. Certified Nutritional Therapy Practitioners (NTP) are trained to perform a functional evaluation and lingual neural testing. These methods are tools to help confirm or deny the efficacy of a supplement. This is an excellent approach to create a bio-individually accurate protocol. Other effective methods may also be available.

Note: Gluten Tolerance Therapies - Gluten Sensitivity Vaccine: According to Green (2016) Nexvax2 is an injectable vaccine designed to induce immune tolerance to gluten. It is designed to work like an allergy shot. It is in clinical trials as of this writing. Other potential therapies include Blocking Tissue Transglutaminase, the enzyme that changes gluten into a toxic molecule for people with Celiac disease; Modifying Wheat; and Bugs as Drugs (Hookworms), and oral Passive antibody therapy. (Green, 2016) These are potential therapies at this time. Your Physician should be your source for information about these therapies if you are Celiac diagnosed.

Chapter 3

What is Gluten & Where Can You Get It?

"How can a nation be great if its bread tastes like Kleenex?"

~Julia Child

Gluten -- [is a] protein composite found in the heart of the grassy grains… (Murray, 2014). Glutens are the major storage proteins of wheat and cereal grains (wheat berries, durum, emmer, semolina, spelt, farina, faro, graham, KAMUT ® khorasan wheat and einkorn), rye, barley and triticale – a cross between wheat and rye. (https://celiac.org/live-gluten-free/glutenfreediet/what-is-gluten/) The main classes of gluten include gliadins and glutenins which are high molecular and low molecular weight proteins respectively. (Lau, 2013)

Gluten acts as a glue to hold food together. It helps foods maintain their shape by giving it structure.

Gluten is used as a stabilizer, flavor enhancer or thickening agent in other food products…. And it's in products you wouldn't expect. (Murray, 2014)

Table 1 on the next page portrays many commonly consumed foods which contain gluten.

Meat, poultry and eggs are regulated by the United States Department of Agriculture (USDA) and don't have to adhere to FDA gluten free labeling guidelines. (Murray, 2014) While we wouldn't find gluten in meat, poultry and eggs by themselves, processed and deli type meats and poultry products may contain gluten.

Table 1: Common foods which often contain gluten. This list isn't meant to be all inclusive.

Soup	Couscous	Pasta*	Sauces
Salad dressings	Food coloring	Malt products**	Cereal
Brewer's yeast	Beer***	Bread	Granola
Brown rice syrup	Lunch meat	Pumpernickel	Crackers
Starch or dextrin	Candy	Soy sauce	Baked goods****
Meat substitutes	Candy bars	Flour tortillas	Breading/coating
Self basted poultry	Multi grain chips	Granola bars	Croutons
Communion wafer	Licorice	Energy bars	Stuffing

*Pasta: including ravioli, dumplings, gnocchi, ramen, udon, chow mein, egg and soba noodles made with only a % of buckwheat flour

**Malt products: including malted barley milkshakes, malt syrup, malt vinegar, malt flavorings, malted milk

*** Beer: Including ale & lager

****Baked goods: Including muffins, bagels, donuts, rolls, croissants, pita, naan, cornbread, flatbread, cakes, cookies, pie crust and brownies

Table 2 offers some gluten product substitutions with non-gluten containing grains..

Table 2: Common Non-Gluten Containing Grains. This list isn't meant to be all inclusive.

Millet	Quinoa (a seed actually)	Rice*
Teff	Montina	Buckwheat**
Amaranth	Oats***	Sorghum

*Brown, White & Wild Rice

**Buckwheat is often combined with gluten grains. Be sure buckwheat products are 100% buckwheat.

***Oats do not naturally contain gluten, but they are often grown in close proximity to gluten grains and /or processed in mills alongside gluten grains leaving them vulnerable to cross contamination. People who eat oats may complain of symptoms which may or may not be due to the oat's exposure to gluten grains. Some people are intolerant of the fiber in oats and/or may have an immune response to oat protein that is similar to a gluten response. When a person has digestive or immune system issues digesting oats, restoring digestive function to optimal may be supportive to be able to eat and assimilate them without issue. Certified gluten free oats are available.

Non-Food Sources of Gluten

Lip, skin care products and shampoo/conditioners must be verified because they are in contact with skin. Everything you put on your skin is quickly absorbed into the bloodstream. Lips, underarms and the scalp are particularly vulnerable, where the skin tends to be thinnest. Manufacturers aren't required to list all product ingredients on labels. It is important to contact the manufacturer if labeling isn't explicitly gluten free. Product labels that include 100% of ingredients are rare. Choose safely by doing your research and looking for gluten free labels on products which come in contact with skin.

Play dough: Although (hopefully) not ingested, children may eat with their hands therefore transferring play dough gluten to their mouth. Washing hands and surfaces thoroughly is important to support the avoidance of cross contamination. Gluten free play dough is available.

Vitamins, herbal and other nutritional supplements may contain gluten. Gluten free labeling of these supplements is now common. Supplements are not regulated by the FDA but they must comply with the Food Allergen Labeling and Consumer Protect Act (FALCPA) which requires manufacturers to clearly list common allergens on their packages including wheat. The same rules apply for 'gluten free' labeling as with food. (Murray, 2014) Cross contamination possibility and listed allergens should also be identified on vitamin, herb and supplement labels.

Alcohol and wine made from a distillation process even with gluten containing grains are said to not contain gluten because the gluten peptide doesn't transfer through the distillation process.

Beer, ale, lager, and malt beverages made from gluten grains are not distilled and are not gluten free. The selection of gluten free beer and cider is growing on store shelves and in bars, making it easier to find gluten free options. Alcoholic beverages with 7 percent or more alcohol and malt beverages made with barley and hops are exempt from FDA gluten free regulations. (Murray, 2014)

Pharmaceuticals: Speak with your Physician to assure medications do not contain gluten.

Chapter 4

History of Eating in America

"You are what you eat so don't be fast, cheap, easy or fake."

~Unknown

America is several generations into a Standard American Diet (SAD) renowned for food products dominated by long ingredient lists and less real food than artificial preservatives, chemicals, and derivatives not designed by nature to feed the human body. Many people do not know much about their food other than recognizing and choosing boxes and packages of their favorite varieties of laboratory made concoctions.

As the American tradition revered as SAD persists, many people have not learned basics of human nutrition and how or why we should feed ourselves real food. Here 'real food' is defined as food that shows up on the plate as close to possible as it is found in nature. Real food isn't highly processed, refined or adulterated. For eons of time some processing, milling or preserving such as fermentation has been done for many foods to be consumed. Traditional methods of processing, milling and preserving food enhance their viability as food, while providing nourishing fuel to energize, grow, restore and repair the human body. Contrary to modern methods of processing, refining and adding preservatives, traditional methods enhance a food's nutritional viability.

Sometimes packaged and processed foods contain real food ingredients although they are usually dominated by artificial preservatives, chemicals and derivatives of food unrecognizable to the human body. The idea of *A Fresh Wellness Mindset* is to choose foods without added artificial ingredients as much as possible. These are foods where the food doesn't have an ingredient label because the food is the ingredient label. Think apples, berries, green beans, fresh wild fish, eggs… you get the idea.

Keeping it real in America, most of us can't and don't necessarily want to be so regimented that we don't eat anything processed, ever. Eating some processed and packaged foods is part of living a modern life with a primary occupation other than growing, raising and preserving your own food. It is easy to learn to make the best choices of the food supply available, wherever you live; and however much you want to invest in your food from a time and money perspective.

Center your food choices around 'ingredient label free foods'; and then augment with packaged and processed foods comprised of ingredients 'as close to nature as possible'. You can make the best choices for yourself when you are a diligent label reader. When you cannot pronounce ingredients on the label or don't know what 'that' is (can't identify the plant or animal from which it originated), you know you're holding a manmade concoction. Manmade concoctions in food can confuse your body, resulting in unwanted and confused bio-chemical reactions. Your body craves stability to well-perform its trillions of functions daily.

Of course, we aren't going to unravel the SAD situation by traveling back in time to when procuring food was nearly a daily proposition. Nor will we go back in time when someone in a household, usually a woman we call Mom, invested many hours every day to preparing family meals. What we can do is make simple and easy choices with *A Fresh Wellness Mindset*. Simply ease into making more real food choices, one meal at a time. You will better your health and the health of future generations when you improve the nourishment of your body. Others will naturally learn by your example of healthful choices.

While you are learning to turnaround the trend of a common food system dominated by unreal food alongside increasing prevalence of illness, there is much to learn from the past. Let's take a look how humans have procured food over many millennia up to today.

Around 40,000 years ago ancestral man hunted and gathered his/her food. This was a daily proposition of searching for food and then using all parts of the animal for food or other life needs. Nuts, seeds, berries, all provided by nature in seasonal cycles were gathered. Societies of people foraged for animals and plants. What they hunted and gathered was determined by seasonal aspects of Mother Nature's offering, and would have varied based on their locale.

The Agricultural Revolution, also referred to as the Farming Revolution or Neolithic Revolution, signified the development of agriculture as an industry. Having been dubbed the Neolithic Revolution, this evolution having taken root around 12,000 years ago, triggered a significant change in society and the way people lived. Traditional hunter-gatherer lifestyles, followed by humans since their evolution, were swept aside in favor of permanent settlements and a reliable food supply. Out of agriculture, cities and civilizations grew, and because crops and animals could now be farmed to meet demand, the global population rocketed—from some five million people 10,000 years ago, to more than seven billion today. (https://genographic .nationalgeographic.com/-development-of-agriculture/)

Not until about 10,000 years ago did societies in Southwest Asia (the famous Fertile Crescent) begin to cultivate and domesticate plants and animals. Food production took over to such an extent that, in the past few hundred years, only an estimated 5 million people have subsisted by foraging. (http://hraf.yale.edu/ehc/-summaries/huntergatherers) On a planet of over 7 billion people, the number of foragers is small in comparison.

Refined sugar was introduced about 400 years ago. It was reserved as a treat for the elite. Producing refined sugars such as packaged white sugar was an expensive and labor-intensive process and therefore only available to the rich. There are stories of commoners blacking out their teeth with charcoal to mimic the rich people's decayed teeth. No verifiable reference was found to this, but it is an interesting story of human nature and if accurate, my how things have changed.

The Industrial Revolution began in the mid to late 1700s and signified the invention of automation in processes including farming and related machinery. This advancement allowed for more food to be cultivated while the population shifted to occupations away from food production. Increased urbanization and greater personal wealth also occurred. British merchant Peter Durand made an impact on food preservation with his 1810 patenting of the tin can. (https://www.thoughtco.com/history-of-the-can-and-can-opener-1991487) Commercial food preservation followed shortly thereafter and signified the beginning of the commercial food industry we have today. The Industrial Revolution is thought to have occurred until the early to mid-1800s.

In the mid-1800s Louis Pasteur discovered heating milk destroyed bacteria. At the time, infection from foods, particularly milk, was a large concern. Mortality from eating contaminated food and milk was common place. Pasteurization also destroys vitamins, enzymes and other nutrients. Today pasteurization is common practice for milk, other dairy products and juice.

Late 1800s: It was from the fruit of Johnny Appleseed's trees that Orrville, Ohio, resident Jerome Monroe Smucker first pressed cider at a mill he opened in 1897. He also prepared apple butter, which he sold from the back of a horse-drawn wagon. (http://www.jmsmucker.com/smuckers-corporate/smuckers-history)   What a treat it must have been for people of this era to enjoy fresh cider and apple butter. Today the Smucker's® brand is on coffee, dog food, peanut butter, cooking shortening, packaged bread dough, pancake mix and more. Crisco® and Pillsbury® are two of the famous and wildly successful J.M. Smucker's ® brands still on store shelves.

Until the 1900s foods were preserved by fermentation techniques or manipulated with the use of yeast. Hybrid plants were produced by natural breeding of related varieties of plants. "Classic selection' using Gregor Mendel's genetic theory was engaged to manipulate and improve plant species.
(http://americanradioworks.publicradio.org/features/gmos_india/history.html)

1900s: Another American food giant, the Kellogg brothers, began their empire in the 1900s. They forever changed the way Americans eat breakfast. (http://www.kellogghistory.com/history.html) Kellogg's® continued to change and add new products including on-the-go cereal bars, crackers, croutons and cookies. Marshmallow Treats® and Pop-Tarts® are two of their many successful brands.

The J.M. Smucker Company and Kellogg Company are two of the earliest food companies in the United States. Their desire and achievement of their American dream began with what must have been noble pursuits. Not only have they employed and fed millions of people over the many decades, but they also played an integral social and economic role in the evolution of the country. With the convenience of readymade food, more women who traditionally stayed at home with the job of feeding their families with homemade provisions have been able to have careers for purposeful work that is very much a part of America. Commercial food preservation, processing and manufacturing has been a cog in the wheel to bring a food supply home in a modern society. Many companies have followed in the actions and success of these two companies.

In the mid to late 1930s Weston A. Price, DDS, traveled the globe for nearly 10 years in search of the secret to health. He focused on healthy people, to find what was in common. He found that although diets varied a great deal, there were native commonalities to all diets in which people were healthy. Dr. Price identified healthy people by characteristics of their physique, facial and dental arch development.   He observed perfection of health in those groups of people who ate their indigenous foods.   He found when these people were introduced to modernized foods, such as white flour, white sugar, refined vegetable oils and canned foods; signs of degeneration quickly became quite evident. Dental caries, deformed jaw structures, crooked teeth, arthritis and a low immunity to tuberculosis become rampant amongst them. (Price, 2014)

Considering that World War II began in 1939, the beginning of the J.M. Smucker Company and Kellogg Company may have been a factor of survival for soldiers during World War II. Soldiers fighting an overseas war needed shelf stable food. New food preservation techniques employed by the new food companies played a vital role.

World War II also signified the invention of DDT. This was important because this was the first U. S. war in which insects and diseases killed fewer people than bullets and bombs, presumably due to the invention of DDT. (http://livinghistoryfarm.org-/farminginthe40s/pests_01.html) The DDT invention paved the way for the discovery of more chemical insecticides, fertilizers and other chemicals to be used in farming and ultimately food production.

Late 1980s to early 1990s: The first field tests of genetically engineered or genetically modified organisms (GMO) crops (tobacco and tomato) are conducted in the United States. Calgene's Flavr Savr tomato, engineered to remain firm for a longer period of time, was approved for commercial production by the US Department of Agriculture. The FDA declares that genetically engineered foods are "not inherently dangerous" and do not require special regulation. (http://americanradioworks.public-radio.org/features/gmos_india/history.html)

Today the proliferation of more food products preserved with artificial ingredients and chemicals, and agriculture and farming techniques engaging genetic engineering have led to GMO crop domination in America. Today GMOs are estimated to be in 75-80% of our food. (http://fortune.com/2016/07/31/gmo-labeling-bill/) This has been propelled by the companies who advance it under the heading of 'sustainability' and a need to feed a growing population. Power arguments abound in media and press channels on the topic of GMO crops.

In the human quest to sustain ourselves, the idea of humankind surviving life by eating primarily unreal food and genetically altered food prevails in our food supply and culture. The power of the media and advertising plays into this scenario as unreal food and drink is promoted and made popular with connotations of athleticism, stamina, beauty, physique, love and popularity. The popular portrayal of health and beauty promoted by marketing and advertising is also big business. The messages conveyed, reflecting great times and happy healthy people fueled by adulterated food aren't realistic for life.

The human body doesn't process manmade chemicals, additives, preservatives, enhancers and altered food well. Ever try consistently watering a plant with soda; or filling your fish tank with artificially flavored and sweetened iced tea from a can; or filling up your car with pudding or plant fertilizer or even diesel when it requires unleaded gasoline? Yes it's ridiculous! But come on, the analogy of trying to feed and fuel something (or someone) with a product it wasn't designed to use as fuel demonstrates the ridiculous idea of humans not eating real food we were designed to eat.

Making better choices need not be overwhelming. It is best for your body when you ease into a better way of nourishing yourself gradually. Easy consistent changes become habits for a lifestyle that creates real health and vitality. Even with advanced, modern busy lives full of activities, work, educational and life pursuits your ancestors might barely imagine, there is much you can do for yourself to simply bring back real food and restore bodily function. You can reap vast rewards real food is designed to provide. Choosing (real) food you love and loves you back is a heartfelt choice to fuel your body for life.

Chapter 5

Be Your Own Wellness Advocate

**"You really have to love yourself to get
anything done in this world."**

~Lucille Ball

In order to have *A Fresh Wellness Mindset* you must be your own wellness advocate. No one should care more about your well-being than you do. Regardless of the status of your health or how near or far you are from making choices healthy for you, have firm resolve to make choices aligned with your well-being. Any action you take with consistency for your best interest can be the beginning of living with greater vitality and health.

A Fresh Wellness Mindset isn't a call for perfection ascribed by someone or something outside of you. Everyone has within them the knowledge to choose in their own best interests. Decide you are going to make choices which feel the best for you and do it.

Going with the best feeling choices isn't about isolating yourself from the input of others. Wisely gather information from a variety of quality sources. New information gives you new ideas and inspiration. Not all the information you gather will resonate as truthful for you. Disregarding something that may be right for others but isn't right for you is empowering. Wellness is about choosing common sense.

When it comes to implementing dietary and lifestyle changes, make simple choices. Simple choices make it easier to isolate what is working and what isn't working. The phrase 'slow and steady wins the race' exemplifies a lasting course for wellness. Now you are moving to a life of greater wellness for your life, so bring in change nice and easy. Many circles say 21 days is the time it takes for change to become habitual. Give your body time to adapt.

While feeling good is always the goal, sometimes a change kicks up a reaction in the body. Sometimes the body adjusts to change by sending you more symptoms like what you are trying to eliminate. Sometimes you may have an allergic or sensitivity reaction which results in rashes, hives, etc. and you need to cut back or discontinue that change. Sometimes a healing reaction can cause you to feel a little worse before you feel better. If you have extreme reactions or anything of concern, consult your Physician or qualified practitioner.

The power of belief is foundational for creating lasting results. The human body is designed for wellness. Anything done for greater alignment to nourish the body with appealing real lively food is of benefit toward healthy function. Firmly believing the power of your body's desire to restore itself to improved wellness is required to feel better.

Belief must be accompanied by action. Even if you are at the farthest point possible from eating healthfully and/or experience symptoms of malfunction, small improvements practiced consistently will move you to improved health. Rather than ascribe another's concept of what to eat, drink and how to enhance wellness with lifestyle choices, learn to make choices that feel right for your body.

Be mindfully aware of what you are eating and drinking. You might think, I am eating this sandwich and drinking this glass of lemonade. A sandwich and lemonade and everything else you eat hold so many possibilities for being a healthful choice or an unhealthful choice. Your meal could be loaded with all kinds of nonsense, nonfood, chemicals, preservatives, and derivates creating havoc for your digestion and blood sugar and offering calories and little real nourishment (vitamins, minerals, protein, healthy fat, and other nutrients) or it could be rich in nourishment offering a source of energy to rejuvenate you and gracefully fuel your body for several hours at least.

Become curious about how your food and drink came to be; where it was grown or raised and what it actually is. Tuning in to whether or not your food and drink is provided by nature or manufactured in a factory is a starting point to considering how well your food is working for you. Whether or not your food has the components of vitamins, minerals and the breadth of nutrients your body is designed to thrive on; or as a means of calories to fill an energetic gap is the difference of nourishment for replenishment and fueling for what is ahead or not.

Read Labels: Look past marketing claims ['natural', 'nothing artificial', 'made with…' etc.] and head straight to the ingredient list of the packaged foods you are considering. If you can't pronounce something or know it isn't grown or raised by Mother Nature, it isn't real food.

Ingredients on labels are listed by their dominance in the product. The most prominent ingredient is at the top and on down in proportion to its inclusion. It is especially helpful to see where sugar falls in the ingredient proportions. Sometimes sugar will be listed several times on a label. For instance, a chocolate chip cookie may have sugar in a variety of forms and also be listed again as an ingredient in the chocolate chip.

One teaspoon of granulated sugar equals 4 grams of sugar. (https://www.webmd.com/food-recipes/features/sugar-shockers-foods-surprisingly-high-in-sugar) When you see a label with 12 grams (for instance) of sugar per serving, it has 3 teaspoons of sugar. Be sure to note the serving size for an accurate picture of how much sugar you are ingesting.

When I began my conscious wellness journey one of the first things I did was to eliminate everything with hydrogenated ingredients. Hydrogenated ingredients are in many commercial food products. Their elimination was a big undertaking and didn't happen overnight. I found hydrogenated oils in bread, nut butter, margarine, canned soups, canned sauces; powdered mixes; frozen potatoes; other frozen food; macaroni and cheese, etc. It can feel frustrating when you learn that foods you have relied on contain unsafe ingredients.

Overwhelm does not do a body or mind any good. Choose one thing; do it well; and progress. Gradually but surely replace what isn't serving you with better choices. In my example with bread, nut butter, margarine, canned soups, canned sauces; powdered mixes; frozen potatoes; other frozen food; macaroni and cheese, there are selections on the shelves without the 'bad stuff' for all of these. To find them you'll have to do some label reading. Going to a naturally oriented grocery market can help because you'll have already eliminated the common big commercial brands which tend to be loaded with the 'bad stuff'. Don't assume because you are shopping in a natural or 'whole' store that everything meets your needs for no chemicals or whatever you begin targeting. Even there, read labels before you put items in your cart.

Leaning in to real lively food begins to transform you. Soon you won't be reliant on packaged products. You'll find making soup from scratch and freezing some for another week is easy. You'll find that making 'oven fries' from scratch is worthwhile and more delicious than the brand you used to go to. Everything you wish to eat has a real lively food counterpart. Soon you won't even consider less than the 'real thing' for you. Balance your resources of time with your desire for real (yummy) food and won't miss your old standbys at all.

Nutritional uptake soars by eating fresh food as much as you are able. Making small sustainable choices consistently is the key to create lasting healthy habits with big positive impact. Make choices suitable for your resources of time and budget while prioritizing for your health status.

When the 'enemy' is gluten, prioritize and remove all products with wheat and other gluten grains. Chapter 10 will be your detailed guide to 'Navigate Life Free of Gluten'. 'Gluten replacement products' are often overwhelmed with chemicals and other non-food ingredients, extra sugar and unhealthy fat to replace the structure gluten provides. You will find more satiation and nutrition when you choose food free of gluten without ingredient labels and discover or make really good substitutes for bread and other baked goods now off limits.

Once you are successfully avoiding the obvious enemy such as wheat/gluten or other food linked to health issues, pick something additional which resonates with you, that you can learn to avoid. Often you only need to pay attention to what your intuition / gut feelings are telling you. Instincts are remarkably intelligent.

Ideas of what to avoid beyond hydrogenated or partially hydrogenated ingredients include: High Fructose Corn Syrup (HFCS); anything hydrolyzed or otherwise not recognizable as grown or raised in nature; and sugar in many of its forms (keep reading for a list of those disguises).

Cross contamination means ingredients may have come in contact with wheat or other gluten containing grains from the machinery, tools or through airborne means. Food labels may refer to 'manufactured in a facility which processes wheat or other gluten containing grains (or other common allergens)'. Labeling disclosures can help identify where cross contamination might have occurred. Allergen labeling is encouraged but not mandatory. (Murray, 2014) When you think cross contamination may expose you to unwanted foods, choose another food to meet your needs.

Sugar: Even with the notoriety sugar is receiving as an ingredient to be avoided, most Americans consume way too much sugar. Sugar promotes unhealthy inflammation, the precursor to dis-ease. More is written in Chapter 6 about how sugar overwhelms and degrades the body's function. In Chapter 6 you'll also be able to read about how much added sugar is likely okay.

Sugar is added to so many common foods. You must be product savvy. To help you identify added sugar in food, use this table as a guide to see how sugar is disguised. Soon you will be able to spot it 'a mile away.'

Table 3: Common names of sugar and its derivatives (not meant to be all inclusive):

High Fructose Corn Syrup	Fruit juice (& concentrate)	Crystalline Fructose	Turbinado Sugar	Maltodextrin	Sorbitol
Date Sugar	Glucose	Honey	Xylitol	Ethyl Malt	Sucrose
Mannitol	Glucose Solids	Diastic Malt	Diatase	Date Sugar	Lactose
Invert Sugar	Caramel	Barley Malt	Carob Syrup	Cane Sugar	Maltose
Dextrose	Fructose	Corn Syrup	Beet Sugar	Agave	Coconut Sugar

Table 4: Common places for sugar in everyday unreal foods (not meant to be all inclusive):

Baking Mixes	Ketchup & other Condiments	Salad Dressings	Luncheon Meats & Bacon	Canned Fruit	Bread, Bagels, Donuts, Baked Goods	Cheese Dip
Nut Butter	Soup	Frozen Vegetables	Yogurt	Hot Dogs	Prepared Seafood	Crackers, Cookies, Bars

Gluten Free Labeling

When you are looking for products to replace gluten containing items, gluten free labeling is a very good thing. Gluten free labeling helps you hone in on minimal ingredient breads (free of gluten), condiments, soup or luncheon meats and so many other items where you wouldn't consider it to have gluten.

According to the Food & Drug Administration (FDA), if a food contains wheat starch, it may only be labeled gluten-free if that product has been processed to remove gluten, and tests to below 20 parts per million of gluten. With the enactment of this law on August 5th, 2014, individuals with Celiac disease or gluten intolerance can be assured that a food containing wheat starch and labeled gluten-free contains no more than 20ppm of gluten. If a product labeled gluten-free contains wheat starch in the ingredient list, it must be followed by an

asterisk explaining that the wheat has been processed sufficiently to adhere to the FDA requirements for gluten-free labeling.
(https://celiac.org/live-glutenfree/glutenfreediet/sources-of-gluten/#O823Tu1EBeHUHJgG.99)

The FDA states, this new federal definition standardizes the meaning of "gluten-free" claims across the food industry. The rule also requires foods with the claims "no gluten," "free of gluten," and "without gluten" to meet the definition for "gluten-free."

(http://www.fda.gov/NewsEvents/Newsroom/PressAnnouncements/ucm363474.htm)

It is worth mentioning again that simply choosing 'gluten free' products to replace bread, crackers, cookies and other common gluten containing products can be worse for the body. Not only do processed gluten free products contain lots of manmade chemicals, derivatives, sugar and unhealthy fat designed to replace the structure that gluten provides, but they are also more costly than real food or gluten containing counterparts.

Here is your guide to labeling icons common in today's grocery market place:

The most common gluten free certification is 'Certified Gluten Free' by gfco.org

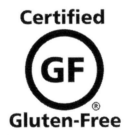

Less common is the Celiac Sprue Association's label. This organization is found at csaceliacs.org

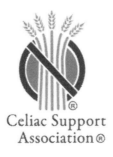

USDA Organic labeling

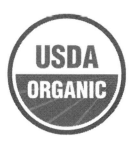

USDA organic products have strict production and labeling requirements. USDA organic products must meet the following requirements: Produced without excluded methods, (e.g., genetic engineering, ionizing radiation, or sewage sludge); Produced using allowed substances; Overseen by a USDA National Organic Program-authorized certifying agent, following all USDA organic regulations. (https://www.ams.usda.gov/rulesregulations/organic/labeling)

According to the USDA, if you make a product and want to claim that it or its ingredients are organic; your final product needs to be certified. A complete list of USDA-Accredited Certifying Agents can be found at https://organic.ams.usda.gov/Integrity/.QAI/Quality Assurance International, OCIA/Organic Crop Improvement Association, CCOF/Certification Services LLC, OTCO/Oregon Tilth Certified Organic and CDA/Colorado Department of Agriculture are some of the more common certifying organizations. If the certifier isn't on the package it isn't certified. If a product provider is not certified, they must not make any organic claim on the principal display panel or use the USDA organic seal anywhere on the package. They may only, on the information panel, identify the certified organic ingredients as organic and the percentage of organic ingredients. (https://www.ams.usda.gov/rules-regulations/organic/labeling)

NON-GMO Labeling

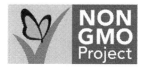

The Non-GMO Project is a mission driven nonprofit organization offering a third party non GMO verification program. Since 2010 they have pioneered industry standards for non-GMO verifications. (https://www.nongmoproject.org/product-verification/)

According to Consumer Reports (https://www.consumerreports.org/-cro/2014/10/where-gmos-hide-in-your-food/index.htm) all of the products they tested with the Non-GMO Project label qualified as non-GMO products. The product had no more than 0.9 percent genetically modified organisms. (In EU countries, products that have ingredients that contain more than 0.9 percent genetically modified organisms are required by law to carry GMO labeling.) The Non-GMO Project certifies manufacturers' products through third-party testing.

Consumer reports went on to say that Uncertified non-GMO claims made by the manufacturer—which may include the words "No GMO" and "Non-GMO"—have no standard definition and don't require independent verification.

In July 2016, President Obama signed a bill requiring labeling of GMO ingredients. The bill isn't satisfactory to all proponents of GMO labeling as they cite it isn't stringent enough (called the DARK Act – Denying Americans the Right to Know). The bill allows companies to use QR codes or an 800 number for GMO labeling. American food companies say it is too expensive to add GMO labeling although 64 countries currently require labeling of GMO products. (http://fortune.com/2016/07/31/gmo-labeling-bill/)

The use of genetic engineering, or genetically modified organisms (GMOs), is prohibited in organic products. (http://blogs.usda.gov-/2013/05/17/organic-101-can-gmos-be-used-in-organic-products/) When choosing whole gluten free grains and rice pasta, always choose USDA Organic & NON-GMO. In 2012, Consumer Reports found measurable levels (of arsenic) in almost all of the 60 rice varieties and rice products (they) tested. (http://www.consumerreports.org-/cro/magazine/2015/01/how-much-arsenic-is-in-your-rice/index.htm)

The USDA Organic label also assures GMO engineering has not been part of the food's origination. Having just the USDA Organic would suffice to assure NON-GMO means, although many foods have both labels. USDA Organic and NON-GMO do not address gluten content.

Natural Labeling

Here's what the FDA says about using "natural" terminology on food labels: Although the FDA has not engaged in rulemaking to establish a formal definition for the term "natural," we do have a longstanding policy concerning the use of "natural" in human food labeling. The FDA has considered the term "natural" to mean that nothing artificial or synthetic (including all color additives regardless of source) has been included in, or has been added to, a food that would not normally be expected to be in that food. However, this policy was not intended to address food production methods, such as the use of pesticides, nor did it explicitly address food processing or manufacturing methods, such as thermal technologies, pasteurization, or irradiation. The FDA also did not consider whether the term "natural" should describe any nutritional or other health benefit. (http://www.fda.gov/Food/GuidanceRegulation/GuidanceDocumentsRegulatoryInformation/ LabelingNutrition/ucm456090.htm) The word 'natural' on labels doesn't have to mean anything. It doesn't relate to a product's gluten content.

Center your food life on 'Food Free of Gluten'. Rather than searching out foods with gluten free ingredient labels, consider choosing 'food free of gluten'. The food is the ingredient. Choose properly grown and raised real food from its natural environment. Think fresh fruits, fresh vegetables (including root and cruciferous veggies, and lots of leafy greens, etc.), grass fed meat, wild fish, wild game, dairy, nuts, seeds, legumes & gluten free whole grains (lots more on this later) and healthy fats (like grass fed butter, extra virgin olive oil, coconut oil, duck fat, grass fed tallow, etc.). Read Chapter 11 & up level your life with real food (zero ingredient labels).

Repeat after me: When I choose 100% real food, the food is the only ingredient.

You Can Do This!

Find Happy Balance: Be your own wellness advocate by finding balance between as perfect as you can get square meals and allowing yourself to flow without the pressure of being perfect.

When you find this happy balance:

- ❖ You aren't looking for a reason to binge out or sneak junkie food upsetting to your equilibrium.
- ❖ You naturally gravitate to food and meal choices that fit for your time schedule.
- ❖ Food doesn't stress you out.
- ❖ Food replenishes you.
- ❖ Food brings you joy.
- ❖ Food is guilt free.
- ❖ You never ever feel deprived where food is concerned.

❖ You get what you need and want.

❖ You feel perfectly satisfied.

❖ You go to sleep satisfied... Not hungry and not guilty for something you ate or drank.

Ingredients are the answer to eating food that seems too good to be true. Choose pizza, ice cream, cheesecake, chocolate anything, pudding, cookies, or anything else, when you want it, provided it is comprised of real food ingredients your body finds appealing. For your body, appealing also means digestible. If you aren't digesting gluten or dairy or anything else well you must avoid it.

Set yourself up for satisfaction. Satisfaction isn't the same as feeling stuffed. Satisfaction occurs when your body has signaled you that the food you are eating is giving satisfaction. You want to slow down naturally, not just because the food is all gone or you feel uncomfortable. Real food ingredients trigger your body to be satiated and nourished. When you are nourished, your body is getting what it needs.

Once you are eating the best real lively food you can afford the vast majority of the time and assimilating it well, you won't want junkie food anymore. A while back I was moving. You know, the week of sandwiches and inevitably a fast food restaurant rears its ugly head. I had been pulling the bun off my chicken sandwiches and eating a few fries. I was feeling deprived and exhausted. I decide to 'treat' myself to a diet soda. I enjoyed diet soda as part of my daily ritual many years earlier as a staple in college and as a regular afternoon indulgence during my corporate career years. The soda tasted awful! After the second sip my body assured me that this was gross. I tossed it. Taste buds reset as they were designed to signal you when your body is becoming nourished. Taste buds will tell you when a food isn't right for you. Rely on the 'taste bud test' when you have been off the junkie food and your body function is working well.

Expansion is the key to evolve your wellness mindset. Continue to learn about the input that fuels your body to thrive. Keep trying new real food. Keep trying new ways of being food-ready with your busy life. Food is vital for wellness, yes. However, even perfect food choices won't do your body any good without great function. Really listen to what your body has to say by the expression of your feelings.

The more you care for yourself at a deep level of seeking nourishment and energy from what you put in your body, the more you will crave what's good for you. Eating right involves a whole lot of common sense and listening to your inner being. Getting in your wellness anyway, your body will give you messages to make choices which honor you deeply. It becomes common sense. Listening and minding the messages of your body is foundational to be your own wellness advocate.

Chapter 6

Unreal Food

"Don't eat anything your great-grandmother wouldn't recognize as food."

~ In Defense of Food author,
Michael Pollan

Food is Information: Choosing real food is an investment in your health, offering improvement to the way you look and feel. What you eat today has an impact on health today, tomorrow and years in your future. Brogan (2016) says food is indeed information.... and we must move away from the notion that food is just calories for energy ("fuel") or that food is simply micronutrients and to come. Choosing A *Fresh Wellness Mindset* becomes easy, delicious macronutrients ("building blocks"). Food is meant to provide energy for our cells in the form of vitamins, minerals, fiber and phytonutrients, that when broken down to a molecular level the body will assimilate for energy, growth and repair. Brogan (2016) goes on to say that food is a co-evolutionary tool for epigenetic expression. Food and lifestyle investments create wealth of health for years and satiating. You won't ever go back to self-destruction.

Several generations of Americans have been surviving on the Standard American Diet (SAD), known for being full of processed and overly refined food. This is food made in a laboratory. People aren't made in a laboratory. We need real food, grown in nature, the 'old fashioned way', the way great-grandmother or her mother did it. Many of us, raised on SAD, have never learned how to put meals based on real fresh food together. Maybe you can make a meal or more than one meal comprised of real food, but if you are like most Americans, you don't sustain yourself that way day in and day out. Instead, Americans largely rely on packaged this and packaged that, fast food and restaurant meals and sugary laden beverages disguised as coffee, tea and even water. It's easy to get caught up in busy modern life. It's ᴄᴀ.. to be lured by enticing food product labels and claims. It's easy to love the idea of food so fast you'd think we've bounded into the times of the Jetson's. But the thing about the Jetson's is they look closer to robots than humans.

Driven by the infusion of non-food ingredients largely making up our food supply, American taste buds have become warped. Bodily function, reliant on real food nutrition, is jeopardized with the intake of laboratory engineered food. Left unattended, this will be a personal health crisis. Many would argue this already is a national health crisis, considering the increasing prevalence of not only Celiac but many modern diseases like Cancer, Diabetes, Alzheimer's and Heart Disease, all rampant in America.

Let's take a look at what is lurking in the ingredient label laden food dominating grocery shelves and dominant in SAD.

GRAS – Generally Recognized as Safe: I used to think, I have no idea what *THAT* is, but *'they'* wouldn't allow it in food if it were dangerous. The 'powers' do allow all kinds of ingredients in food arguably not in the best interests of those who consume it. Leading my list of these ingredients is something called GRAS – Generally Recognized as Safe. According to the FDA, GRAS is any substance that is intentionally added to food is a food additive, that is subject to premarket review and approval by FDA, unless the substance is generally recognized, among qualified experts, as having been adequately shown to be safe under the conditions of its intended use, or unless the use of the substance is otherwise excepted from the definition of a food additive. (https://www.fda.gov/Food/IngredientsPackagingLabeling/GRAS/)

GRAS guidelines can't take into account bio-individuality including how much a person is consuming or what happens with extended consumption over many years. While a serving size of a GRAS ingredient may be deemed to be 'safe', people may consume larger quantities and multiple products with the GRAS ingredient. Functional issues such as digestive troubles, auto-immunity or another condition may strengthen a weakness for dealing with GRAS ingredients.

According to *Consumer Reports* (https://www.consumer-reports.org/food-safety/gras-hidden-ingredients-in-your-food/), 'In all, there are an estimated 1,000 GRAS substances for which safety decisions were made by the food industry without any notice at all to FDA, and thousands more chemicals for which both proof of safety and continued federal oversight are minimal.' *Consumer Reports* goes on to say, some GRAS-designated substances, like trans-fats and mycoprotein or Quorn (a meat substitute made primarily of fungus), have been the subject of high-profile criticism and other GRAS substances even suspect of being possible carcinogens. "FDA missed a major opportunity to clean up the food system," says Laura MacCleery, vice president of Policy and Mobilization for Consumer Reports. "Companies will still be able to introduce novel substances into food in secret, without having to show they are safe. The agency also failed to fix the rampant conflicts of interest that affect the review process for ingredients."

Avoiding food with unpronounceable ingredients and catch all phrases like 'natural flavoring' are a good way to avoid GRAS ingredients. If you don't recognize an ingredient as being grown or raised in nature, chances are it is laboratory made and may be on the GRAS list.

Excitotoxins: Since the inception of the first food manufacturers, processed food has become inundated with manmade chemicals, additives and derivatives tricking the brain to over consume it. These chemicals cause food to appeal to your sense of taste in a way that is not authentic for your well-being. Unreal food hijacks the brain to keep eating without satiation. See this in your own life when in one sitting, the last cracker in the bottom of the box tastes as good as the first one. And make no mistake in understanding excitotoxins aren't limited to crackers. Excitotoxins are in packaged snack foods, baked goods, luncheon meats, soups, sauces, mixes and many food products. Unreal food becomes 'junkie food' when your brain is tricked to overconsumption.

Excitotoxins make up many of the manmade chemicals added to food. Their artificiality is another means by which your brain is hijacked. You can't seem to get enough. You eat more. Food manufacturers sell more products. Monosodium Glutamate (MSG) is one commonly used excitotoxin added to food as a flavor enhancer. Excitotoxin consumption leads to overconsumption. Dr. Blaylock, says "These (excitotoxins) are substances, usually acidic amino acids, that react with specialized receptors in the brain in such a way as to lead to destruction of certain types of neurons." (http://landofpuregold.com/the-pdfs/Excitotoxins.pdf) Our brain is signaled to keep on eating while neuronal destruction occurs at a subtle level. One may think to avoid 'MSG' on a label, but the tricky thing is, excitotoxins are able to be in products under other labeling names such as natural flavoring/ flavoring/ natural flavor(s), hydrolyzed vegetable protein; autolyzed protein, plant protein, textured protein, yeast extract, anything with glutamate, nutritional yeast and carrageenan. For your brain not to be hijacked by 'junkie food', commit to only choosing food with ingredient labels where you clearly know what the ingredients are.

Other common excitotoxins are aspartate (aspartame), domoic acid, cysteine and L-BOAA/ODAD.

With practice and consistency avoiding excitotoxins, your taste buds relearn and crave real food. You will eat to a point of satiation, as the body signals you it is fulfilled with nourishment. Healthy cravings will find you when you convert to real food. Listening to your body's wisdom, real food satisfies you. More about cravings is in Chapter 12.

Frankenfoods: Controversy whether GMO foods are Frankenfoods is plentiful. Frankenfoods could be extended to include GMOs because of the manipulation standpoint around GMOs, but Frankenfood and GMOs are two distinctly different categories of food to avoid. GMO foods are more difficult to spot because they also appear as fruits and vegetables in their whole form.

Consider Dr. Mark Hyman's definition of Frankenfoods. According to Dr. Mark Hyman, "The biggest problem about demonizing a food substance is when the food industry manipulates "Frankenfoods" by removing ingredients and adding other bad stuff instead. As 'gluten free' gains popularity, food companies – well aware of a potential marketing opportunity – turn regular junk foods into 'healthy' gluten free versions. Don't be fooled. It's still junk food. … read its ingredients: Those types of products are usually higher in sugar, flours (that converts to sugar), inflammatory fats like vegetable oil, and weird foodlike additives that add up to big profits for these companies and added padding around your midsection while sabotaging your health." (http://www.mindbody-green.com/0-28707/could-going-gluten-free-cause-inflammation-a-doctor-explains.html?utm_source=mbg&utm_medium=email-&utm_content=daily&utm_campaign=170228)

Frankenfoods are made with adulterated ingredients manufactured in a laboratory. If they originated in nature these ingredients have been manipulated by the food company beyond recognition of their original design. The simple common-sense way to understand the nonsense these ingredients impart on the human body is that the human body wasn't designed to be fueled on artificiality or synthetic anything. I come back to the argument of watering a plant with something other than water or putting something other than the proper gasoline in a gas engine. When you feed something with a substance other than what it was designed for it won't run efficiently or at all or it is headed for a breakdown.

Modern Wheat & White Flour: These are Frankenfoods in their own right. Given the problem of their indigestibility leading to conditions like Celiac and blood sugar dysregulation, they deserve their own paragraph. Ill grown (chemically treated) grains are further damaged by modern methods of extreme processing. Commercial milling finalizes their death sentence. Their economic favorability (cheap) and need to feed an enormous population has propelled their inclusion in an enormous variety of packaged food. They deserve a place as a major contributor of a failed food supply.

Pollan (2008) refers to white flour as the first fast food. Void of nutrition, except for the synthetic nutrition pumped back in during the manufacturing process, the processing these flours undergo also depletes fiber. This big zero will likely tamper with blood sugar regulation because it quickly turns to sugar in the body and may not be well digested. Undigested foods are left to ferment and potentially be seen as a foreign invader by the body (auto-immunity may result).

Sugar. Sugar dominates ingredient labels. Take a peek back to Table 4 in Chapter 5 to be reminded that sugar lurks everywhere. Indeed, it does lurk because it is often disguised (see Table 3 in Chapter 5 for many common names under which sugar and its derivatives hide).

Americans consume around 130 pounds of sugar every year. Our 1822 predecessors ate under 10 pounds of sugar a year. 130 pounds a year means about three pounds a week. That equals about 3,550 pounds in an average lifetime—approaching two tons of sugar. Imagine an industrial dumpster with 1,727,900 skittles and you've got 130 pounds of sugar. (http://www.alternet.org-/food/9-shocking-facts-you-need-know-about-sugar) Or if it is easier for you to get the visual, pile three pounds of sugar in front of you and imagine actually eating all that sugar this week. This 'average number' of three pounds of sugar consumption each week is even more shocking if you consider many people don't eat near this much sugar so others are eating much more. I've done some informal surveying of people on the topic of sugar consumption. I reveal the shocking statistic of sugar consumption to be average 3 pounds a week. Never once has anyone said, yeah, that sounds about right. The people I have 'surveyed' are people in my life who I know eat a lot of common sugary foods, processed foods and aren't reading labels. They say something to the effect of the quantity of sugar consumption is ridiculous; and they certainly aren't eating that much sugar. But I would bet they are eating that much sugar and maybe more. They just don't know it because they aren't reading labels, don't know how to decipher what they see on labels (sugar disguises and how many grams = one teaspoon of sugar). Don't be a victim to consuming too much sugar. Know what is in your packaged and processed foods and you will be taking a big stride to preserving your health.

The truth about sugar!

- ❖ Sugar is addictive. It releases opiate like substances which activate the brain's reward system.
- ❖ Sugar creates a blood sugar roller coaster contributing to hyperactivity, mood swings and Diabetes.
- ❖ Sugar suppresses the immune system. Some say sugar is cancer's favorite food.
- ❖ Sugar contributes to Candida (yeast overgrowth - a yeasty foamy white bug (lives in your gut) like activity feasting on your sugary processed foods and drink.
- ❖ Sugar contributes to nutritional deficiencies. It is a big zero and takes up space for what otherwise nutritional food would nourish and energize your body.
- ❖ Sugar ages the body.
- ❖ Sugar can cause a 'hangover' effect including fuzzy or foggy thinking, fatigue, gas/bloating/extended stomach, headache/migraine, joint pain, constipation, diarrhea, skin problems, allergy symptoms.

Sugar is implicated as a causative factor in heart disease, cancer and diabetes as well as the obvious issue of obesity. In a study done by the *Journal of the American Medical Association Internal Medicine (JAMA Intern Med)* it was concluded that 'Most US adults consume more added sugar than is recommended for a healthy diet. We observed a significant relationship between added sugar consumption and increased risk for CVD (Cardiovascular Disease) mortality.' (Yang, Zhang, Gregg, Flanders, Merritt, & Hu, 2014).

Exactly how excess sugar might harm the heart isn't clear. Earlier research has shown that drinking sugar-sweetened beverages can raise blood pressure. A high-sugar diet may also stimulate the liver to dump more harmful fats into the bloodstream. Both factors are known to boost heart disease risk. (http://www.health-.harvard.edu/blog/eating-too-much-added-sugar-increases-the-risk-of-dying-with-heart-disease-201402067021)

Oncology Nutrition (https://www.oncologynutrition.org/erfc/-healthy-nutrition-now/sugar-and-cancer/) states "Much research shows that it is sugar's relationship to higher insulin levels and related growth factors that may influence cancer cell growth the most, and increase risk of other chronic diseases."

Eating refined sugar is calorie consumption without fiber, vitamins, minerals or other nutrients. Too much sugar consumption can deplete minerals. Sugar consumption contributes to dental cavities and crowds nutritious food out of the diet.

Here is something American Heart Association® has gotten right: They recommend women consume less than 100 calories of added sugar per day (about 6 teaspoons) and men consume less than 150 (calories of sugar) per day (about 9 teaspoons). (http://www.heart.org/HEARTORG/HealthyLiving/HealthyEating/HealthyDietGoals/Sugars-and-Carbohydrates_UCM_303296_Art-icle.jsp#.WMM_6qPrvIU) To put that in perspective, a 12-ounce can of regular soda contains about 9 teaspoons of sugar, so quaffing even one a day would put all women and most men over the daily limit. (http://www.health.harvard.edu/blog/eating-too-much-added-sugar-increases-the-risk-of-dying-with-heart-disease-201402067021)

Begin removing Unreal Foods. For every serving, sip or bite of unreal food you remove you will immediately be doing your body and mind a favor toward wellness. Foregoing unreal foods will boost healthy blood sugar regulation for heart health, cancer prevention, happy stable mood and more (see above).

Be diligent. With consistent practice of removing one unreal food at a time, your body will display a cascade of healthy benefit. It takes about 21 days for behavior to become a habit. Starting in a gradual fashion will show you positive rewards and it can be nice and easy for the body. When you support one small positive behavior, your body will begin to reset and restore itself. If you are eating more than one of these (and most Americans are), start with one, the easiest one and consistently avoid it for 21 days. Replace it with a real food or beverage, as a delicious satisfying replacement. Repeat.

Common American (unreal) foods to forego for better all around wellness:

❖ **Soda, diet or regular, all soda** is loaded with ingredients that are not good for the body or mind. Soda has neurotoxins which are destructive to nerve tissue. Soda contains aspartame (an excitotoxin). Drink half your body weight in ounces (if you weigh 150 pounds, drink 75 ounces) in pure water every day to flush the bad and help the good flow. Idea to replace: Purified water, iced or hot herbal tea, kombucha, kefir, coconut water and fruit kvass. Add fresh fruit slices to water or drink fruit essence infused water (read labels on bottled options to be sure you aren't getting more sugar).

❖ **Canned and bottled teas or other drinks with long unpronounceable ingredients**
See above. It is usually filled with all kinds of sugar or other junk. Idea to Replace: It's easy to put a tea bag in water and make tea – iced or hot. It's delicious and fresh.

❖ **Yogurt with any form of sugar.** The sugar destroys good benefits of the yogurt. Choose whole fat plain yogurt, ideally from grass fed cows or other pastured animals (goat, sheep). Idea to Replace: Whole milk grass fed yogurt, coconut yogurt or almond milk yogurt.

❖ **Nut butter with any ingredient other than nuts.** These are loaded with toxic hydrogenated oils, other refined oils and sugar. Idea to Replace: Organic and no sugar or extra oil added nut butters are available.

❖ **Processed Cereals.** These are extruded (a process in manufacturing) that destroys nutrients. Idea to Replace: Quinoa porridge, homemade granola or soaked gluten free oats with real fruit and nut toppings. Add a dash of honey or maple syrup if more sweetness is desired.

❖ **White/modern wheat bread.** Soft, pliable, chewy, white flour and chemical laden bread creates havoc with blood sugar regulation. Idea to Replace: Choose organic and bread free of gluten (read the label for minimal whole real food ingredients). If gluten isn't an issue and digestion is strong choose bread made from organic and sprouted gluten grains. Learn to bake sourdough from quality grains. Eat less bread! (See Table in Chapter 10 for bread/gluten grain replacements)

❖ **Fancy coffee drinks with unknown ingredients.** Burned old pesticide sprayed beans and chemical laden additives and ingredients are what you often get from coffee conglomerates or others. Idea to Replace: Freshly (locally) roasted beans and cold brew or use a French press.

❖ **Catsup with High Fructose Corn Syrup (HFCS) or other sugar.** This highly refined processed corn is probably made from GMO corn. Ingredients aren't real food. Idea to Replace: Make your own catsup with organic tomatoes, vinegar, onion, honey or choose an organic brand made without HFCS and other unwanted ingredients.

❖ **Condiments with sugar** in any of its forms. Idea to Replace: Read labels to choose products made without sugar and unidentifiable/unreal food ingredients.

❖ **Chips with sugar and chemicals.** Read labels to see what you are getting with sugar, unhealthy oils and other unreal ingredients. So many of these compressed food particle 'chips' are worse than potatoes. With potatoes or other veggie chips at least you can recognize the food. Idea to Replace: Choose chips as a 'cheat treat' made in coconut oil (safe at high heat) and organic potatoes or other vegetables like beet or sweet potato chips. Dehydrating food is easily done at home with a dehydrator. Kale chips are easy to make and nutrient dense.

❖ **Low fat anything.** The fat is replaced with sugar and chemicals to make the food taste normal. Your body needs fat as nature provides. Fat often shows up with quality protein. Quality protein and healthy fat work together in the body for energy and strength. When you forego the fat you will forego protein naturally and eat more food that converts to glucose quickly. Idea to Replace: Salad dressings made from olive oil and lemon juice; Bake up a 'paleo' cookie or bar recipe for a snack with lasting energy; Dips make with sour cream and yogurt will satisfy you; Choose hummus from chickpeas, beets, and parsnips for dips.

❖ **Juice Drinks.** The pulp and fiber are removed along with many important nutrients whole fruit provides. Juice quickly turns to glucose in the body, spiking blood sugar. Idea to Replace: See #1 above.

Chapter 7

Body Works

"All disease begins in the gut."

~Hippocrates (the father of modern medicine)

The human body is entirely purposeful. Trillions of bio-chemical reactions and functions are synchronized as if the body is an amazing machine or orchestra presenting a complex piece. Each reaction and function relies on one and another to transform your food into energy, vitality, thinking ability, rejuvenation, restoration and growth.

Body function can be categorized into large groups which represent the trillions of tiny reactions taking place. Digestion and blood sugar regulation are much of the focus of this book. More major system function includes the immune system, lymphatic system, urinary system, reproductive system, endocrine system, cardiovascular system, respiratory system, integumentary (skin) system, muscular system, and the nervous system(s). Small sustained change is remarkably rewarding because when improvement is seen in one system function it is natural for other functions to improve.

Structure of the skeletal system also supports the functional design and vice versa. The miracle of bodily function goes barely recognized by the human being until something isn't working so well. Until then, many humans rationalize and negotiate with themselves that the little tiny signs and symptoms are normal. While one headache, a rare bout of digestive trouble or something else so randomly miniscule may not be something worthy of delving into its source, the recurring signs and symptoms the body expresses are reflective of burdened function.

Homeostasis is the scientific term for balance the body constantly strives for. When the slightest trigger or stressor (think minor temperature change) occurs, the body adapts. You don't usually feel homeostasis at work even though it is the foundation of your body's design. Homeostasis allows the body to give and take, providing more support to the highest priorities as functional burden occurs.

You may not feel the effects of too much stress, not enough sleep, a processed and refined diet, or eating the wrong foods for you right away. The body amazingly compensates for stressors. The body is trying to tell us something with the little signs and symptoms which become bigger and louder. Pick any malady and you can relate it to earlier signs and symptoms. Most adaptations by the body go unnoticed by your senses until uncomfortable signs and symptoms show up.

External havoc is a reflection of internal disorder. Unhealthy inflammation creates chaos with function and the body's quest for homeostasis. Then comes breakdown of optimal function and you realize you may be in trouble if you don't do something different. Earlier attention invested in how you feel can intervene to turn back signs and symptoms.

As with the mechanics of a machine, when something starts clanking, if it isn't fixed, the clank (symptom) will progress to inefficient function at best and perhaps breakdown all together. Caring for the human body's signs and symptoms need not be burdensome though. And chances are, the sooner you look into the source and do something about it the easier it is to fix.

I know this to be true from my own life. I rationalized genetics were the source of my body's complaints. I didn't want to slow down my life to really pay attention and get to the bottom of it because I didn't have the information I am sharing with you. Had I tuned in to my body earlier and simply known the signs and symptoms were reflection of burden I could relieve, I wouldn't have had to feel so much pain and invest so much of my resources of time and money to unravel what led to something that could have stopped me in my tracks.

Wherever you are with your wellness status, food can be a major contributor to wellness and improving your health. Wisely tuning in to know which choices are healthy for you as a unique person and then taking action in the direction of healthy choices is a beautiful notion. Lifestyle (like stress management and sleep) and thinking and motion are more ways we can support wellness.

As with food, it is important to make lifestyle adaptations and improvements that are healthy for you. Different amounts of sleep, stress relief, relaxation and exercise are right for each possible. You must honor the needs of your unique body in all areas of living for optimal wellness.

The term 'Functional Food' sounds like a weird science project. In reality, 'Functional Food' is really yummy, satisfying real food. It is readily abundant and easy to bring into your modern busy life. You may invest as much or little time as you prefer to center your food life on Functional Food.

Functional Food at its best is simply done. I can't emphasize how easy it is to eat food that is really good for you once you know which choices are healthy for you. As you get in the groove with food which serves you really well, you won't think functionally. You will naturally gravitate to foods personally appealing. The way to make this happen in your life is described in detail in Chapters 12 and 13.

If Functional Food sounds distasteful, too scientific or anything other than joyful, it isn't being done right. By nature's design, real food is the answer to hunger. Real food miraculously fuels the entire spectrum of human bodily function.

Satiation is one of the greatest benefits of choosing real (functional) food without an ingredient label. Without satiation, we are plagued by one of the most prevalent health detriments - insatiable eating. Over consumption is famous for making people over weight. When we over consume, we eat more calories (the energy factor of food) than we expend in motion to burn all of the calories. We tend to over indulge in carbohydrate rich food like crackers, chips, cookies, donuts, etc.

These foods quickly turn to glucose, the body's form of blood sugar. The body can't use all the sugar ingested from carbohydrate rich and other sugary foods. Glucose the body does not use immediately is converted to glycogen as the storage form of glucose. Excess blood glucose is stored as fat and triglycerides. The CDC says, more than one-third (36.5%) of U.S. adults have obesity. Obesity-related conditions include heart disease, stroke, type 2 diabetes and certain types of cancer, some of the leading causes of preventable death. (https://www.cdc.gov/obesity/data-/adult.html)

Healthy satiation is achieved when blood sugar regulation is normalized by quality protein and healthy fats balanced with real food carbohydrates like lots of colorful non-starchy vegetables. Veggies and whole fruit add complex carbohydrates with vitamins, minerals, fiber and phytonutrients to your nutrition uptake. Long burning sustained energy will happily take you from breakfast to lunch (and lunch to dinner), giving your pancreas a proper rest from chronic insulin release. Ideally a 12-14 hour fast from dinner to breakfast will give the digestive system a rest.

Blood Sugar Regulation: Every time we eat, insulin is released by the pancreas to facilitate the uptake of glucose into cells for fuel or storage. With chronic overconsumption, or day and night long grazing on food, the pancreas can become worn out or unable to release insulin effectively. When the body isn't releasing or utilizing insulin correctly, the result may be the onset of Type II Diabetes or insulin resistance. According to the Centers for Disease Control and Prevention (CDC), 'From 1990 to 2009, the rates per 100 of diagnosed diabetes in the United States population increased by 217% (from 0.6 to 1.9) for those aged 0–44 years and by 150% (from 5.0 to 12.5) for those aged 45–64.' (https://www.cdc.gov/diabetes/statistics/prev/national/figbyage.htm)

It is nearly impossible to over consume processed and highly refined modern wheat products and not create imbalanced blood sugar leading to unhealthy blood sugar patterns. All sorts of maladies show up as hyperglycemia and hypoglycemia evidenced by headaches, fatigue, moodiness, energy issues, glycation (advanced aging) of cells, insomnia and more. Blood sugar issues are often evidenced by the need to eat frequently (every couple of hours) with other feelings of emergency needing to be compensated immediately with food. A Physician or qualified practitioner can test blood sugar levels for accurate numbers indicating blood sugar patterns and stability to guide you to restoration.

When blood sugar is unsteady, healthful real food choices (quality protein, healthy fat, mostly non- starchy veggies and whole fruit in moderation) are especially important selections and should be eaten as needed to maintain equilibrium. Juice drinks and sugary foods should be avoided. Even though whole fruit is abundant with vitamins, minerals, other nutrients and fiber, since it is often higher in sugar content than other real food, limit whole fruit to one piece or less per day to support restoration of steady blood sugar levels.

Working with your nutritionally trained Physician or other qualified practitioner can help you make choices to restore optimal function. When blood sugar regulation is normalized you can build on healthy benefits for longer burning energy. Healthy benefits are being able to have a daily mini fast from dinner to breakfast, better digestion, sleep, natural detoxification and rejuvenation. Less snacking between meals also lessens the need to stock up on expensive snack foods and you won't have to tote food everywhere you go!

Digestion begins in the brain with a cascade of internal triggers signaling food is coming. The brain begins to prepare the body to receive the food. When you've felt your mouth begin to salivate because the sizzle of a steak (or some other wonderful real food) fills the room or approaches the dining table, digestion is beginning. 'Pre-digestion' happens when you smell a big pot of Grandma's recipe for tomato sauce, a hearty stew, homemade chicken noodle soup or homemade sourdough bread baking (or other delicious concoction of real food ingredients).

Salivation is good. Imagining your favorite real foods, you may begin to experience a natural pre-digestive response of the body. The brain is telling the body to begin producing digestive enzymes. Properly chewing food efficiently reduces it to a paste-like or nearly liquid form in the mouth. The mechanical action of the teeth and tongue break down the food into a liquid paste the esophagus and stomach receive. Adequate chewing effectively releases salivary amylase which is necessary for carbohydrate digestion.

The stomach releases more digestive enzymes with the power to turn a sizzling steak or plate of raw greens into liquid. This enables the pancreas, small intestine, liver and gallbladder to do their jobs of emulsifying and assimilating the meal's nutrients. When liver and gallbladder function is compromised, bile won't be released for fats to be emulsified. Emulsified healthy fat is required for the important vitamins A, D, E & K to be absorbed in the body.

More than 90% of nutrient absorption takes place in the small intestine. When food isn't properly broken down in the digestive process, Auto-Immunity can begin in the small intestine, where food intolerances, allergies, Celiac disease and NCGS can be borne. Further down the digestive chain of events is the large intestine's function to recycle some nutrients and eliminate the waste. Undigested carbohydrates left to mingle in the large intestine can contribute to dysbiosis, yeast overgrowth and other maladies of the large intestine. Elimination of waste can be impeded, leaving toxins to stay in the body.

When digestion isn't working well, you can become malnourished because your body isn't breaking down your food to nutrients it can absorb and assimilate into energy for life. If you aren't properly digesting, even the best food can cause discomfort. Undigested food is of no benefit to us and can actually do harm, as in the case of Celiac and other Auto-Immunity. Even eating the best real food can lead to food intolerances, sensitivities or allergies. Undigested proteins putrefy; fats become rancid; and carbohydrates ferment when not digested.

Supporting optimal digestion is a force fundamental for expression of wellness. Optimal digestion may overcome some food sensitivities. I've seen it in my own life with eggs, tomatoes, gluten and more. Optimal digestion enables your body to receive benefits of nutritious real food. The body wisely knows how to convert food to energy for immediate use, store energy for future use, move nutrients in and out of cells, repair tissues, bones and muscles, rejuvenate you after a stress event or busy day, and naturally detoxify you from the onslaught of environmental, food, water and product toxicity.

Take Hippocrates, quote 'All Disease Begins in the Gut' for practical benefit and acknowledge optimal wellness also begins in the gut.

Tips to boost your digestive power and support optimal digestion:

❖ Add ¼ tsp fennel seed to warm water and drink 20 minutes before meals.

❖ Or add some lemon juice (a wedge or teaspoon) or apple cider vinegar (start with ¼ tsp and work up to teaspoon) to an eight-ounce glass of water 20 minutes before a meal. Note: Don't take fennel, lemon and ACV at the same time. Just try one that resonates with you.

❖ Eat in a calm and relaxed state. Ever heard the phrase 'Rest and Digest'? It's true... the body only digests food when we are calm and relaxed.

❖ Sit down when you eat.

❖ Avoid eating in the car (unless you are having a blood sugar need and this is your best choice).

❖ Make the meal time table as pleasant as you are able. Adding nice placemats, dishes, clearing anything not meal related... whatever you care to add for pleasantries sends your brain loving messages and brings you to a place of beauty and peace.

❖ Turn off the TV.

❖ Don't discuss stressful situations or problems at mealtime.

❖ Turn off your devices during meals.

❖ Don't listen to the news during a meal.

❖ Take a break. Enjoy the food and people you are dining with.

❖ Put on some relaxing music.

❖ Be purposefully grateful for the meal.

❖ Notice the meal's appearance, smell and beauty.

❖ Give yourself at least 20 minutes to enjoy and savor a meal. 30 minutes or more is better!

❖ Admire the texture of the food. Chew food until it is a paste, and the paste becomes a liquid. This requires more than four chews and a gulp. Being mindful helps. Pay attention to what you are eating and when you are swallowing. Count bites if you must - this is important.

❖ Drink only a little water or other liquid with your meal and for a while (45 – 60 minutes) thereafter. 4 ounces is adequate to help you swallow the food. The digestive system doesn't like to be flooded out. Too much liquid dilutes precious digestive enzymes. A little water is good with meals.

❖ If you wish to try digestive enzyme supplements, seek the advice of a qualified practitioner (such as NTP) to test efficacy of a professional line and find out the right dose. Each body is different. Supplements are not created equal. Testing helps you choose wisely for your body and your wallet. Poor quality supplements can be detrimental.

❖ Don't eat for 12 – 14 hours after dinner until breakfast. This mini-fast will support complete digestion of the last meal of the day, pancreatic function, natural detoxification, restoration and rejuvenation (best sleep) for your body. Note: If you are restoring blood sugar regulation, you may need to eat more frequently. If this is you, compensate with a protein based snack.

The foods in Table 5 on the next page are especially supportive of good digestion. Optimal food choices will vary for each person. Avoid anything which creates distress or is unappealing.

Incorporating as many of these foods into your diet on a regular basis which you find appealing may assist your body with digestive function. Improved digestion increases how well your body is able to assimilate foods for absorption of nutrients for energy creation and the trillions of other functions your body performs. Incorporate new foods gradually so as to not overwhelm your body.

Table 5. Foods to support digestion. This list isn't meant to be all inclusive.

FOOD	IDEA
Apple Cider Vinegar	A small amount in water 20-30 minutes before a meal may assist in protein digestion.
Beets	Especially good for purifying blood. Support the liver, a key player in digestion. High in fiber. Good source of manganese for pancreas. Juice, roasted, grated on salads, cultured.
Cabbage, garlic, onions, leeks	Sulfur rich veggies support glutathione production which is a chief antioxidant for the liver, also support insulin. Anti-parasitic. Roasts, sauté, juice the cabbage, culture/ferment.
Ginger	Stimulates saliva (release digestive enzymes), relaxes and soothes digestion. Grated on veggie dishes, pickled before a meal, added to smoothies.
Dandelion Root	Supports bile flow, Good prebiotic - contains inulin. Use the root as a tea, or make a salad of the leaves.
Bone Broth	Contains glycine and collagen, both good for digestion. Sip & Enjoy, Use as the liquid in rice or quinoa dishes.
Lemon	Added to warm or room temperature water is a good digestive tonic first thing in the morning or 20 – 30 minutes before meals.
Fennel	Said to tone and strengthen the stomach, soothes intestinal pain, spasms or cramps. Enjoy raw, steamed, baked. Added to soups and stews. Use instead of celery in recipes.
Pineapple	Contains bromelain which is anti-inflammatory, protein digesting, high in manganese for pancreas. Supports small intestine. Eat raw or lightly grilled or sautéed.
Apples	The pectin in apples is a soluble fiber that may improve the intestinal tract's ability to eliminate waste. Eat raw or baked with skin. Eat a variety of cultivars.

Radish	High in vitamin C, said to support the flow of bile (due to high sulfur) and thus good for liver, gallbladder and digestion. Enjoy a variety of cultivars raw.
Celery	High in natural fiber and water. Natural mineral salts bond with trace minerals and nutrients to support good enzymatic activity. Enjoy celery juice in the morning as a digestive tonic.
Jicama	Low glycemic root vegetable high in fiber. As a prebiotic, jicama is good food for probiotics in your gut. A juicy in season jicama tastes similar to an apple. Eat raw, grate on salads or prepare like oven fries. Don't eat the seeds or skin.

Lymphatic Flow: Restoring digestion includes supporting lymphatic flow. The lymphatic system is an integral part of the immune system. According to the National Institutes of Health (NIH), the lymphatic system has three primary functions. NIH says: "First of all, it returns excess interstitial fluid to the blood. The second function of the lymphatic system is the absorption of fats and fat-soluble vitamins from the digestive system and the subsequent transport of these substances to the venous circulation. The mucosa that lines the small intestine is covered with fingerlike projections called villi. There are blood capillaries and special lymph capillaries, called lacteals, in the center of each villus. The blood capillaries absorb most nutrients, but the fats and fat-soluble vitamins are absorbed by the lacteals. The third and probably most well-known function of the lymphatic system is defense against invading microorganisms and disease. Lymph nodes and other lymphatic organs filter the lymph to remove microorganisms and other foreign particles." (https://training.seer.cancer.gov/anatomy/lymphatic/)

Contrary to a mindset that eating gluten grains contributes to depression, according to Douillard (2017), 'The real culprit of what has come to be known as "gluten-related depression" is likely due to overconsumption of highly processed refined white flour products and congested lymph channels that drain the brain. Poorly digested gluten can enter the lymph through the intestines and cause lymph congestion.'

Including raw food as part of your daily diet brings high levels of naturally occurring enzymes which serve as catalysts to assist the breakdown of toxins and enabling them to clear from the body. This reduces the burden on the lymphatic system and liver. Fresh fruit and raw vegetables are high in water which aids the body and lymph system with removal of unwanted compounds. The alkalinity of raw food neutralizes harmful pathogens which in turn lessens the burden on the lymph system. Healthy digestion is a pre-requisite for consuming raw foods. Raw food diets aren't right for everyone. Begin with one raw food a day to see how it agrees with your digestion. Add raw foods gradually and go by how you feel.

A qualified herbalist may make recommendations to include cleavers, red clover, manjistha or another herbal remedy to aid healthy lymph flow. Always consult with a qualified herbalist when considering herbs to assure good quality and efficacy for your body's needs.

Hydration is vital for healthy lymphatic flow because lymph is primarily water. Adding lemon to water assists the body with hydration. The alkalinity of lemon helps mineralize the body and lymph. Use a straw (glass or BPA free) to drink lemon water for protection of tooth enamel (or rinse with clear water after drinking lemon water).

Lymphatic flow doesn't 'just happen' as with your cardiovascular or blood circulatory system. Optimal lymphatic function requires stimulation by skeletal movement. According to Northrup (2012), One of the main reasons why exercise has such healing power is that it vastly increases the lymph circulation in your body. To speed up lymph flow she recommends: Don't sit for long periods of time; breathe deeply and regularly; move; avoid over exercise. Taking a walk after a meal and bouncing on a mini-trampoline daily can be restorative and supportive of good lymphatic flow and digestion. Even a few minutes, working up to ten minutes or longer on a mini-trampoline is useful. Dry brushing the skin with a natural bristle brush supports lymphatic flow. Always brush gently and lightly, as if you are petting your pet, from extremities and toward the heart, where lymph is combined with blood after the lymph is cleansed by our lymph nodes. Northrup (2012) describes how a light touch skin self-massage can accelerate the transport of impurities to the lymph nodes for cleansing. Lymphatic massage received from a qualified practitioner is also helpful for lymphatic flow.

Chapter 8

Grains: The Good, Bad & Ugly?

O beautiful for spacious skies / For amber waves of grain / For purple mountain majesties / Above the fruited plain! / America! America!

~ Katharine Lee Bates

Grains often get a bad rap in America. The haranguing of all whole grains is often a botched comparison of the real deal and a laboratory made project. An educated comparison of a truly whole grain like organic rice and overly processed and refined so called whole grain cereal, crackers and bread produces night and day results. The nutrient panel on the processed and refined product may reflect quantity of nutrients, but remember those nutrients are likely to be 'pumped' back in to the final product as synthetic counterparts. The real nutrients of the food ingredients have been milled and processed and extruded leaving a nutrient void bundle of calories and blood glucose spiking product which will leave you searching for sustenance within a short time. On the other hand, organic brown rice (as an example of a real whole grain), comes from nature with B vitamins, manganese, phosphorus, iron, fiber, essential fatty acids, selenium and copper just as nature created.

Eating and properly digesting quality grains in moderation can be a source of nourishment and energy creation for your body when you are adequately digesting and assimilating the grain. Whole grains are fiber rich; have antioxidants, B Vitamins, phytochemicals, minerals, protein, and vitamin E. Refined grains are mainly composed of only the endosperm portion of the grain. When the milling process removes most of the bran and some germ, along with the majority of fiber, vitamins, minerals, antioxidants and phytochemicals, the grain becomes void of nourishment. As much as 75% of phytochemicals (phytonutrients) are lost in the refining process. (http://www.health.state.mn.us/divs/hpcd/chp/cdrr/nutrition/facts/whole-grains.html)

Many of the refined and processed 'whole grain' products have been manufactured at very high temperatures leaving them not only void of nutrition but very difficult to digest. To compound digestive issues, blood sugar spikes and falls cause distress (mood, energy, fatigue, headaches, insomnia etc) and precipitate long term health issues. These product ingredient labels often lead with wheat.

Please don't be misled to think that wheat in its wholesome form as nature provided resembles what you are getting with extremely processed foods. Not only do these foods quickly convert to glucose (blood sugar) in the body, but they often contain sugar in more than one form and unhealthy oils/fats. Excitotoxins, more chemicals, derivatives and preservatives are also ingredients. Manufacturing manipulates any real food ingredients to be a vague resemblance of their original form. These products are not adequate in nutrition to be considered a healthy grain component of a well-balanced nutritionally dense diet.

Humans have been eating grains for thousands of years. That's not to say that truly whole grains are right for everyone in the same quantity. To sort out whether whole grains are right for you and how much is right for you, consider the following:

❖ Is the food truly whole grain or real close to how Mother Nature designed it? (how much processing has it been through)
❖ If the grain is in bread or crackers or another product, take a look at the ingredient list. Is it combined with unrecognizable and unpronounceable ingredients?
❖ How much sugar is added?
❖ Is it organic?
❖ And very importantly, even if your wellness status is in good check to digest and assimilate the grain, *how do you feel* when you eat whole grains?

Source and quality of grains play a large part in how well a person handles the grains. Tips to choose grains wisely:

❖ Choose USDA Organic grains. Grains tend to absorb heavy metals and even arsenic along with the pesticides and fertilizers. Choosing organic is a priority.
❖ Select grains from packages for fresher products than those from bins in grocery stores.
❖ Store grains in the freezer or refrigerator in airtight containers to preserve their longevity.

Those with Celiac or NCGS may find reprieve from having a void of wheat and other gluten grains by incorporating rice or other non-gluten containing whole and good grains into their food life.

Note on Quinoa: Actually a seed, quinoa (pronounced Keen-wah), from a broad leaf plant is a pseudocereal. It works nicely as a gluten free grain replacement. Quinoa cooks much like rice in broth or water, add some veggies if you like and serve it as a side dish. Adding black beans with other chopped veggies (peppers, carrots, onions, broccoli, etc) makes a great easy reheat meal. Serve it up with salsa and top with sliced green onions. Quinoa works as a hot cereal. Serve it with milk of your choice, chopped nuts and fruit. Quinoa is a complete protein, meaning that it offers all of the essential amino acids. Quinoa is fiber rich and has a variety of vitamins and minerals including B vitamins, copper, iron, manganese and phosphorus. It is closely related to spinach and beets.

Isolate your reaction to grains by withdrawing them from your diet and adding back in slowly and in small portions. By slowly, add them one at a time, giving pause for feeling the food's effect on your system. (More on reintroducing offending food in Chapter 9) Even with the best quality properly prepared whole grains, we must balance grains with quality protein and healthy fat for optimal blood sugar regulation.

Some people may feel better eating grains at lunch or dinner while others find it preferable for their body to avoid grains at dinner.   Listening to your body, and the way you feel when you eat food will reveal much. Eating in a calm and relaxed setting supports your awareness to tune in to your body's preferences.

In a diet balanced with quality protein, healthy fat, a wide array of vegetables and whole fruit, begin with 1/8 cup working up to ½ cup serving of a whole grain such as brown rice, wild rice, farro, kasha (whole grain buckwheat), wheatberries or bulgur (cracked wheat). Make the right choice of gluten or non-gluten containing grains for you. Begin with one small serving once a week. When you don't experience digestive or other adversity as a result of one small serving, slowly work up to two and then three times a week. This nice and easy approach gauges how your bio-individual makeup is digesting and assimilating whole grains. Don't consume food offering signs and symptoms of stress on your digestive system.

Government food intake recommendations present a one size fits all approach to tell us what we should be eating.   Grains comprise ¼ of the USDA's Choose My Plate (https://www.choosemy-plate.gov/). The USDA Food Pyramid recommends 6 ounces of

grains daily and half of them whole grains. "Eat at least 3 oz of whole-grain cereals, breads, crackers, rice and pasta every day."
https://www.cnpp.usda.gov-/sites/default/files/archived_projects/MiniPoster.pdf

Such a general statement as this one provided by the USDA leaves grain consumption, be it processed or truly whole grain, completely wide open. One might imagine if their 'at least 3 oz' recommendation means that six ounces or 20 ounces or more is better. According to this recommendation from the USDA you could polish off a couple boxes of excitotoxin laced 'whole grain' crackers everyday and be following your government's recommendation. It just doesn't add up to common sense for health.

Modern processed and refined grains are an easy and tempting choice in a busy life. With the government advice above it may be tempting to justify consumption of food that really doesn't do your body any favor. Just pour cereal and add milk or toast any bread or prepared pastry for breakfast. Mix up a packaged floury (additive loaded) bowl of batter for a treat of pancakes or cake. Grab some 'whole grain' bars, crackers or cookies for a snack but wait a minute. Read ingredient lists and know your body needs real food.

Douillard (2017) writes, "Part of the problem is that we, as a culture have overshot the wheat and gluten runway. The typical American diet has included eating wheat with every meal for the past 40-50 years. We have overeaten wheat in a major way." Wheat, traditionally a seasonal crop, is now available year- round. As with so much of the food supply, this crop was not intended to be eaten year-round and in the quantity now consumed. This issue combined with the quality and over processing of the wheat supply (and other gluten and non-gluten grains) has confused our body and disrupted optimal function.

When you over consume a food, you confuse the body's natural design of balance. Overconsumption of wheat, a food intended to promote the storage of energy for winter, translates to fat & triglycerides. Add in over processed and refined wheat ingredients in many food products, and overconsumption issues are magnified. Overconsumption creates an addictive cycle contributing to blood sugar dysregulation, other digestive issues and health issues like obesity.

Brogan (2016) says that "carbohydrates have been a key to human evolution; and there's no way we could have developed such big brains had it not been for our access to carbohydrates in addition to high-quality protein." The mammalian brain depends upon glucose as its main source of energy, and tight regulation of glucose metabolism is critical for brain physiology. Consistent with its critical role for physiological brain function, disruption of normal glucose metabolism as well as its interdependence with cell death pathways forms the pathophysiological basis for many brain disorders. (https://www.ncbi.nlm.nih.gov/pmc/articles/PMC3900881/) Low-carb diets are not likely to meet the high glucose demands of the brain.

Humans have salivary amylase, the enzyme to break down carbohydrates. Brogan (2016) says that we (humans) have many copies of the genes that code for salivary amylase where as other primates have only two copies. In other words, humans have a much greater ability to digest starch than other primates because we can produce more salivary amylase.

Along with choosing quality sources in moderation, you must thoroughly chew grains and other carbohydrates to aid in adequate release of salivary amylase for digestion and assimilation of nutrients. The majority of carbohydrate intake should be vegetables, particularly non-starchy veggies. Adding in small to moderate amounts of quality, properly prepared real whole grains when digestive function is great, this food can be transformed to 'super' food status.

Brogan (2016) says she has "yet to meet a woman on a long-term low-carb diet who is loving life." After a thirty-day plan resembling the "Paleo diet" Brogan (2016) reintroduces gluten-free grains and beans. Rather than leaving grains in a taboo spot in modern food thought, each person may benefit to find what grain choices suit their unique body.

Whole Grain Nutrition

Now that you know how to sort out real whole grains from 'has been' impersonators, take a look at more nutritional information of the real deal (good quality whole grains):

According to (https://www.hsph.harvard.edu/nutritionsource/whole-grains/):

❖ Whole grains contain bran and fiber, which slow the breakdown of starch into glucose – thus maintaining a steady blood sugar rather than causing sharp spikes.

❖ Fiber helps lower cholesterol as well as move waste through the digestive tract.

❖ Fiber may also help prevent the formation of small blood clots that can trigger heart attacks or strokes.

❖ Phytoestrogens (plant estrogens) and essential minerals such as magnesium, selenium and copper found in whole grains may protect against some cancers.

Whole Grain Stamps (http://wholegrainscouncil.org/whole-grain-stamp)

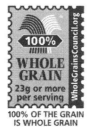
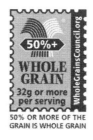
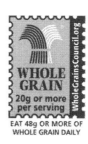

Also according to Harvard's 'The Nutrition Source', (https://www.hsph.harvard.edu/nutritionsource/whole-grains/), one study revealed that inconsistent food labeling means that foods identified as "whole grain" are not always healthy.

❖ The study assessed five USDA guidelines that appear on labels of whole grain foods: any whole grain as the first ingredient, any whole grain as the first ingredient without added sugars in the first three ingredients, the word "whole" before any grain ingredient, a carbohydrate to fiber ratio of less than 10:1, and the Whole Grain Stamp.

❖ The Whole Grain Stamp is a widely used marker on food products. The stamp, while designed to steer consumers toward healthy whole grains, actually identified products that were low in trans fats but higher in sugar and calories than whole grain foods without the stamp.

❖ The other three USDA guidelines had mixed results in identifying healthier whole grain products, but the carbohydrate to fiber ratio of less than 10:1 proved to be the most effective measure of healthfulness. Foods that met this criterion were low in trans fats, sodium, sugar, and calories.

Phytic Acid in Grains: Phytic acid is present in grains, nuts and seeds. While said to be an enzyme inhibitor or anti-nutrient, there is no consensus in the literature regarding mineral deficiencies from a high grain or phytic acid diet. (Douillard, 2017) Fallon and Enig (1999) describe phytic acid as a substance which ties up phosphorus in the bran of whole grains. In nature the benefit (of phytic acid) may be the slowdown of the absorption of sugars after a meal and thus it is found to reduce cholesterol and triglycerides. (Douillard, 2017) Phytic acid is considered by some to create or contribute to digestive difficulty. Perhaps the lesson is that those with more sensitive or stressed digestive function or in digestive restoration mode would be best served to avoid phytic acid or minimize its effects with traditional preparation methods to aid pre-digestion

Sprouting, overnight soaking and old-fashioned sour leavening can accomplish this important pre-digestion process in our own kitchens. (Fallon & Enig, 1999)

❖ Rinsing and then soaking raw nuts and seeds overnight (or for 8 hours) in purified water with a teaspoon of sea salt, rinsing thoroughly and then slowly dehydrating at a low (less than 150 degrees) temperature will support the pre-digestion of the nuts and seeds. The result is even more delicious presoaked and slowly dehydrated than without doing this. When you see what comes off the nuts and seeds you may feel happy you aren't also ingesting this debris.

❖ Rinsing, soaking and re-rinsing rice or other whole grains for eight hours or longer before cooking will also support pre-digestion and a digestive system on the mend. Rice cooks the same, although has a fuller texture when pre-soaked.

❖ When you aren't soaking to minimize phytic acid, giving rice a rinse prior to preparation removes the dust that results from processing and storage prior to packaging.

Spelt, a hardy, high-fiber variety of wheat, has been found to have 40 percent less phytic acid content and more phytase activity when compared to a variety of common wheats. Spelt also had a significantly higher mineral content than most wheats, suggesting that spelt may be much easier to digest and a more nutritious variety of wheat to start with when we reintroduce wheat back into the diet. (Douillard, 2017). Douillard (2017) goes on to say that using the right kind of flour makes a difference in the digestibility of the wheat. Studies have shown that ancient wheat is much simpler, genetically, than modern hybridized wheat.

Sprouting

Sprouted foods contain proteolytic enzymes which help us digest carbohydrates and proteins efficiently. The source cites more efficient digestion with this enzyme activity. (http://www.naturalnews.com/034899_proteolytic_enzymes_metabolism_digestion.html)

According to Fallon and Enig (1999), traditional farming encouraged germination of grains before consumption. The process of germination produces vitamin C and changes the composition of grain and seeds in numerous beneficial ways. Sprouting increases vitamin B content, especially B2, B5, and B6. Carotene increases dramatically – sometimes eightfold.

Fallon and Enig (1999) continue to say sprouting neutralizes phytic acid that inhibits absorption of calcium, magnesium, iron, copper and zinc; and also neutralizes enzyme inhibitors present in all seeds. These inhibitors can neutralize your enzymes in the digestive tract. Enzymes act as catalysts for biochemical processes in the body.

Incorporating sprouted grains is a great way to add a diversity of nutrients to any diet, gluten free or not. A gluten free person who adds buckwheat and amaranth sprouts will add a delicious source of grain nutrition including high protein, fiber, minerals, vitamins and a low glycemic factor (supportive of healthy blood sugar regulation in the body). Buckwheat sprouts offer a mild, nutty flavor. Amaranth is another delicious grain seed when sprouted.

Experimenting with non-grain sprouts adds more high impact nutrition and diversity to your diet. According to Dr. Mercola, 'The vitamin E content, for example (which boosts your immune system and protects cells from free radical damage) can be as high as 7.5 mg in a cup of broccoli sprouts compared to 1.5 mg in the same amount of raw or cooked broccoli.' Dr. Mercola goes on to say 'Sprouts are also an excellent source of fiber, manganese, riboflavin, and copper, along with smaller but significant amounts of protein, thiamin, niacin, Vitamin B6, pantothenic acid, iron, magnesium, phosphorus, and potassium.' (http://foodfacts.mercola.com/sprouts.html) A few non-grain sprouting seeds to try include broccoli, china radish rose, garbanzo and fenugreek.

Choosing Sprouting Seeds

❖ Be sure to choose a seed source offering USDA organic seeds.
❖ Choose a source that sends samples from each lot of seed to an independent laboratory for testing for food borne pathogens.

Almost any grain or seed can be sprouted except for flax and oat seeds. Irradiated seeds will not sprout. Fallon and Enig (1999) do not recommend sprouting alfalfa seeds. They say, it seems that the praise heaped on the alfalfa sprout was ill advised. Tests have shown alfalfa sprouts inhibit the immune system and may contribute to inflammatory arthritis and lupus. Alfalfa seeds contain an amino acid called canavanine that can be toxic to man and animals when taken in quantity. Fallon and Enig (1999) say canavanine is not found in mature alfalfa plants.

Sprouts are delicious on salads, sandwiches, topping for omelets, quiche, frittata, baked sweet potatoes, tacos, wraps and in casseroles. If you can dream of eating it, you can top it with sprouts! Fallon and Enig (1999) warn against overconsumption of raw sprouted grains as raw sprouts contain irritating substances that keep animals from eating the tender shoots.

My recipe to sprout seeds:

What you will need:

1. Sprouting seeds. When combining seeds, choose seeds of about the same size.

2. Quart size canning jar. There are two options for the jar. Either choose one with a ring that you can fit a slightly larger piece of window screen so you can rinse and drain seeds through the screen or a special sprouting jar with a lid that has holes. Sterilize jars and lids (and screen) with boiling water before use.

3. Purified/non-chlorinated or fluoridated water & 1 tsp regular bleach

Step 1 (the extra safety step): Add 1 tsp bleach to 1 cup lukewarm water and soak seeds for 15 minutes. Triple Rinse the seeds and add more lukewarm water. Let soak for 8 – 12 hours.

Step 2: Rinse, gently swirl and drain the seeds a couple of times daily in purified lukewarm water. Leave the seed jar upside down to completely drain in a glass dish, keeping them out of direct sun.

Step 3: Continue this process daily until the seeds are fully sprouted... usually about 7 – 10 days. To remove the seed coats, remove the lid with some water in the jar, hold back the sprouts with a spatula, gently swirl and let the seed coats float out with the water.

Step 4: When sprouting is complete, rinse and drain one last time, remove from jar with very clean hands and utensil and let air dry in a colander in a cool spot on the counter. Use another paper towel to cover your sprouts while they air dry.

Step 5: Store in an air tight container in the refrigerator along with a paper towel to absorb extra moisture. Eat within a few days. If any spoilage is noticed sooner, discard immediately.

Voila! You can easily enjoy nutritious and delicious sprouts made at home.

Kids love to be part of this process.
Children are eager to eat the veggies they grow (sprout) and may develop healthier habits for life.

Sprouts do best in cooler temperatures.

If your sprouts aren't performing in warmer months it may be due to warmer kitchen temperatures.

Chapter 9

Lose Annoying Food & Restore Yourself

"Rest and be thankful."

~William Wordsworth

Figuring out how to support optimal function with food and feel great isn't always too complex. Much of the time, great advancements can be reaped in how we experience wellness by engaging simplicity, mindfulness, real food and nurturing lifestyle practice. Small sustained changes (building new habits easily) equates to nourishing benefits for the body, mind and spirit.

Your food life must be centered on real food, without too many ingredient labels. Too many ingredients and ingredient labels make it more challenging to identify the enemy if unwanted signs and symptoms present themselves. You want to be able to remove what is ailing you. Simple food choices make it easy to peel back the layers, find a culprit and support digestive function. It is much easier to connect the dots to what ails you or creates mischief with function when you are making simple food choices.

Never stop paying attention to how you feel. The premise of personalizing your food life is to feel good. The annoying seemingly small (in the beginning) reactions and stress shows up in your body as your guide. Just because the American culture is abundant with people who are sicker than you or complain of the same things you feel, it isn't normal for your body to be burdened by food. Nip annoying reactions (signs and symptoms) and thoughts in the bud so they don't bloom into an annoying deep-rooted weed.

Digestive signs and symptoms aren't the sort of personal issues most people wish to discuss. It can feel embarrassing to discuss and much less fun to experience. This may seem like all the more reason to want to ignore it and suffer with digestive trouble as gas, bloating, constipation, diarrhea, heartburn, etc. just hoping it will go away. Digestive troubles might also express themselves as rashes, trouble sleeping, headaches, loss of appetite, fatigue etc. Annoying signs and symptoms indicate function is stressed. No matter how you may try to negotiate with yourself, they are NOT normal function.

Beyond the burden to the digestive function (hampering uptake of nutrients from food), food may be distressing function. For instance, when the body isn't digesting gluten, the signs and symptoms appear (refer to Chapter 3) and further gluten ingestion will stress function even more. Damage will continue. Annoying signs and symptoms of any sort will not go away by themselves. Their presence may rise and fall, but they will persist and most likely escalate to greater burden in the body.

Getting on the trail to find the source or root cause of functional issues is important to stomp it out. The reversal of dysfunction, which may implicate dis-ease in the future, is the path to wellness. By now you should have it down that signs and symptoms in the body indicate bodily burden and stressed function. You can do something about it and feel better!

Identify the Offender: If you are still eating sugary, chemical laden Frankenfoods, your first step is to gradually shift to a food life based on primarily real foods. Use the list in Chapter 6 to begin removal of unreal foods in your diet. This might take you a few weeks to more than a few months to make this transition. Your body is designed to begin rewarding you soon with better function and energy. This is a core 'must do' when your body is overwhelmed and expressing burdensome signs and symptoms. You want to feel better and support a path for optimal future wellness.

Real foods annoying to proper function may seem innocent enough because they 'should be' healthy. When digestion isn't working well, even a beautiful salad may cause distress. Even the best food won't provide favor when function is out of order. The food itself may not be the problem per se. The problem is function. There is no way around it: Annoying food must be removed if function is to be restored.

If the 'beautiful salad' is bothering you then try steaming your veggies. Eat just one veggie at a time to know if a specific food is bothersome. Add one healthy fat to one meal in the beginning. A client was stir frying veggies in coconut oil, adding olive oil, sesame oil or flax oil, and sometimes added avocado oil and ghee to one meal. Eating healthy fat is a sound idea, but easy does it. If fat assimilation is burdened, too much of a good thing creates more havoc. Be sure you are using the right fat/right cooking or prep method (see Chapter 11).

Virtually any food can be suspect for a food sensitivity or allergy. Gluten grains are perhaps the most popular or common annoying food, right up there with dairy or casein (a group of proteins commonly found in mammalian milk). Examples of other common annoying foods include tomatoes and other nightshades (peppers, eggplant, potatoes etc), chicken, nuts, soy, strawberries, shell fish and eggs. Annoying foods are often real foods we used to eat without issue.

Once function is restored, sometimes the food may be reintroduced successfully. Each person's tolerance or bio-chemical ability to successfully digest and assimilate reintroduced foods once problematic varies. It takes a combination of restoration of function, bio-chemistry and belief, all of which are bio-individual. When reintroduction isn't possible there are many other foods to eat.

Restoration & Reintroduction

Here's my story: When I was restoring my digestion, blood sugar regulation and immunity; an IgG Antibodies test showed virtually everything (real food) I was eating to be problematic (fish, meat, vegetables, grains and fruit included). It didn't make sense to me that so much food was the problem entirely. I gleaned, for my body's function, already in distress, I needed to eliminate these 'normally healthy' foods and target foods with properties to soothe and restore me.

I had already given up gluten for about six months and thought my diet was good even though I wasn't feeling too much better. It was stunning and quite frankly depressing to receive test results indicating my body wasn't assimilating (and therefore the foods were creating distress) so many common (should be healthy) foods. I worked through it and honored the findings. I ate a limited diet and avoided the problematic foods.

I targeted healing foods like those in Table 5. During that time of a few months, my diet was limited. My perseverance paid off. I was unstoppable because I made up my mind I 'had to' fix my digestive function.

I engaged smart supplementation (tested for efficacy) to restore the integrity of my digestive system along with targeted food choices. I was able to turn my immunity, overall health and digestive system around for good. Now I eat a very diverse diet without adversity. I am excited to share that this year I resumed eating organic gluten containing grains which are properly prepared and in their natural form or close to it (sprouted and soaked). I ate my first whole wheat berries! The first time I ate organic sprouted whole wheat toast after many years of abstinence was nothing short of amazing.

Overall, it has been a journey of months and years to get where I am. The sooner you intervene with your ill feelings, the faster you have opportunity to feel better. The experience of using food to restore me and be able to reintroduce formerly offending food with success has been a blessing. My journey has not been a return to SAD nor will I ever resume eating SAD foods. I am a diligent label reader when I choose a packaged option and I make the vast majority of my food at home, from food without ingredient labels. My food life isn't glamorous although I consider all of my food beautiful. It is simply beautiful because it works for me. When I dine out and travel, I faithfully use the tips offered herein.

Satisfying is delicious. Delicious is satisfying.

Food is meant to be enjoyed. The caveat is you must be eating real food. The 'food stuff' (also referred to in this book as unreal food and junkie food) some people push into their body's system with more resemblance to a scientific project as evidenced by the scientific names on the ingredient label rather than real food grown and raised in nature, really doesn't deserve to be called food (in my opinion).

As defined by *Merriam-Webster*, food is "material consisting essentially of protein, carbohydrate, and fat used in the body of an organism to sustain growth, repair, and vital processes and to furnish energy; also: such food together with supplementary substances (such as minerals, vitamins, and condiments). (https://www.merriam-webster.com/dictionary/food) My point made.

Don't eat food you don't like. When you make something to eat that doesn't turn out to be a favorite, whether it is a new recipe or trying a new food, unless time and money are of no consequence, eat it if it just isn't 'amazing' (Reflecting a preference for not wasting food). Then of course you won't make it or purchase it again.

The differentiator to this scenario and not eating food you don't like is if a practitioner or other source for 'wellness or healing' foods is recommended and you don't like that food, don't consume it. Let the practitioner know that particular food won't work for you and ask them to recommend something else. Food is only 'super-food' when it tastes good for your body and is real lively.

Trying to consume disagreeable food is pointless. You could soon be falling into old unhealthy habits and making unfavorable choices toward unreal food. Leaning in to real lively food you find appealing will help your body and taste palate reset itself for a preference of real food over poor choices. Keep your food life centered on real lively food you love.

There are so many options for restorative foods and foods with a rich spectrum of nutrients. Take a look back at Chapter 7 for a review of so many foods supportive of digestion. Avoid what you don't like. Having *A Fresh Wellness Mindset* is about finding satiating pleasure and gratitude from your body for awesome food.

Rejoice with praise for a beautiful birthday meal such as the perfection of a succulent piece of perfectly prepared fish and seasonal vegetables. Maybe the fish is bacon wrapped shrimp or scallops still sizzling on the plate when served. Think of your best great food experience and make choices in this direction whenever you are able.

The response your body offers to your food is the key to personalize your food plan. Food need not always be a marvelous birthday meal. Joy and a wonderful response from your body should come from all your food. Astonish your body with an amazing apple, crisp fresh produce and nourishing balanced breakfast every day. If your food isn't astounding you it is time to regroup on your choices and slow down when you eat to enhance the experience.

Example: When you begin a protocol such as lemon in water first thing in the morning or before meals, it may appeal to you for a while and even be something you look forward to. You think of your intention of adding the lemon to water as a tonic for your digestion and liver function. You appreciate the crisp zing when you taste the lemon and even imagine you can feel your function perk up with gratitude for this nourishing beverage. But if you don't experience positivity (it makes you squint and clench) of the lemony beverage, either ever or at some point in time, the tonic won't be of benefit to you. This principle can be applied to any food or drink. Finding what you like requires you to be quiet with yourself and let your body agree or disagree with the idea.

The major caveat is when you are shifting from SAD to *A Fresh Wellness Mindset*. Eating SAD, your taste buds are out of sync with what your body really prefers. Because the junkie food comprising the SAD tricks your brain with messages to eat more of the chemically laden food, you only *think* you love SAD food. In reality, this food creates an addictive behavior. When you gradually shift to real food with staying power, your taste buds will reset. In time, you would find the SAD food very unappealing taste-wise (and feeling-wise).

You must return to the way your body was intended to consume, digest and assimilate nutrients from real food to allow your body to support you optimally. Each person is different in the method and means which will be effective to bring back restoration. The investment of effort and resources is worthwhile.

Optimal function is the basis for living and feeling good. Enjoying as many diverse real food choices as possible leads to nutrition meant to support your life. The earlier a person recognizes a functional issue, the 'easier' restoration of function can be. When you intervene what your body is telling you, you can head off health issues for optimal wellness.

If you've been consistently eating a real lively food diet sans known irritants like gluten, and you still have distressing symptoms (or new and advanced symptoms have presented), complicated food interactions or intolerances may be causative. You may be a 'complex case'. Some bodies react adversely to chemical compounds of certain foods. Histamine, oxalates, salicylates, phenols, glutamates, amines, FODMAPS and more may weigh in to the complexities impacting your wellness factors.

Complex cases should engage with a qualified practitioner or Physician who will be able to assess bio-chemistry with laboratory tests; will delve into genetic history; health and lifestyle history; environmental factors including toxin exposures; and invest the time to thoroughly consider your unique deficiencies, excesses and food reactions. A qualified practitioner or Physician will be able to evaluate immunity/auto-immunity; digestive, neurological and metabolic function closely. When you are a 'complex case', your investment of time and resources working with this person may save you resources and health in the longer term than stumbling through pain, discomfort and trying to figure it all out yourself and then feeling no better for it.

Firstly find restoration of function - digestion, immunity, blood sugar regulation or whatever has been ailing you. When signs and symptoms are no longer prevailing, revisit with your Physician or qualified practitioner, any blood work or other tests used to measure your function. When test results confirm what you are feeling, you may want to try to reintroduce the gluten or other food that once bothered you. You must always follow the advice of your Physician. In some instances (Celiac diagnosis or true allergies) you may not be able to reintroduce a food your body has 'rejected'.

The importance of belief in conjunction with the aforementioned indicators cannot be overstated. If you are happy and content without desire to reintroduce a food you once had issue with, then leave it alone. Same goes if you believe a food is entirely bad. There is so much in the media about the evils of gluten, touting all of it as toxic for everyone. When you hold belief a food is all bad, or doubt reintroduction will work, your belief is upheld. The power of our beliefs has a stronghold on how our body works.

I used these tips to reintroduce gluten grains:
I was not tested for Celiac although I used to experience profound digestive pain for a few days if I advertently got gluten in my food at a restaurant. Reminder: Always consult with your primary care Physician or Naturopathic Doctor before making any significant changes to your health and wellness routine.

One Way: Choose a certified USDA organic source. Prepare with time honored (soak or ferment) preparation methods. Begin with one bite. Wait a few days and watch for signs and symptoms that may appear in mood and/or digestion etc. If you are clear of adversity, eat 1/8 cup and wait for a few days and watch for signs and symptoms in mood and/or digestion. Gradually increase serving size to ¼ to ½ cup or the equivalent.

Once you have cleared a grain, wait at least a couple of weeks to reintroduce another as you wish in the same size and controlled fashion, watching for signs and symptoms. Journal your dietary results and intake, pay attention and keep it simple to make it easy to correlate how you are feeling with what you ate.

Another option, if it feels right for you, is to take a quality gluten digesting supplement as advised by a qualified practitioner or Physician before you ingest the gluten containing food. Follow steps above.

Reintroduction of gluten grains when possible is not a return to a Standard American Diet. Successful reintroduction is an uptake of diversity in nutrition and the grain specific nutritional qualities.

If you aren't a candidate for reintroduction, the world abounds with so much beautiful nutritious food. Keep eating and enjoying real lively food you love and loves you back.

Coca's Pulse Test: This is a test that can be easily performed, to use as a tool to help identify food sensitivities.

Coca's Pulse Test is from Dr. Arthur Coca's book *The Pulse Test* that was published in 1956 which is now public domain on the internet. (http://soilandhealth.org/wp-content/uploads/02/0201hyglibcat/020108.coca.pdf) Coca's Pulse Test may be among the easiest methods of food sensitivity testing without special training or expensive equipment. The theory is that food intolerance leaves a stress response in the body causing the pulse rate to increase. The test is not an exact science but may be a helpful tool to confirm food sensitivities.

Full details can be seen in the book and should be reviewed for complete understanding of Dr. Coca's suggested method. Dr. Coca's test directs you to record your diet for 5-7 days and record your full one minute pulse 14 times per day (before rising, before retiring to bed at night, and before each meal and at 30, 60 and 90 minute intervals after each food or meal was eaten). It is important to take your full one minute pulse. Do not take one 30 second pulse and times by two. The challenge for many people would be taking the pulse 14 times per day. With so many diets based on food with ingredient labels it may be more challenging to decipher what ingredient if not a real food by itself causing increased pulse rates.

The LNT Coca Pulse Test is a means to test specific foods rather than the rigorous pulse testing described above that could be difficult to identify specific food sensitivities because you are testing based on meals assumedly comprised of multiple foods and ingredients. There are detailed references available on line for the LNT Coca Pulse Test directions. The summarization is that you will test specific foods for sensitivity based on your pulse rate. If after establishing your baseline pulse, you ingest a small amount of the food, chew it a few times but don't swallow; wait 30 seconds and re-measure your pulse for a full minute with the food still in your mouth you can determine which foods are distressing your body. Coca's theory is if you eat a food you are intolerant to, your pulse will be quickened by six or more beats. The more it rises, the more tension your body is incurring from ingesting the food. The results of recorded pulses can be analyzed in a food journal to determine the foods you are intolerant.

The results may be revealing and helpful for you to disqualify foods from your diet for an elimination period. If you are considering reintroducing eliminated foods retesting your pulse rate can reveal if you have a new tolerance for the food.

I don't recommend these tests as a replacement for consulting with your Physician, Immunologist or Allergist. The tests are a tool which may be a resource for you to research and decide if it is right for you. Always consult with your appropriate Physician or other qualified professional before making changes to your wellness routine.

Food allergies are a serious matter. According to the American Academy of Allergy, Asthma & Immunology, a true food allergy can cause a serious or even life-threatening reaction by eating a microscopic amount, touching or inhaling the food. Anaphylaxis may occur and can be fatal.

(https://www.aaaai.org/Aaaai/media/MediaLibrary/PDF%20Documents/Libraries/EL-food-allergies-vs-intolerance-patient.pdf)

Food allergies must be treated and addressed by a Physician and/or Allergist & Immunologist. Always seek the advice of a qualified expert in this field when you suspect a food allergy may be affecting you.

Chapter 10

Navigate Life Free of Gluten

"You may not control all the events that happen to you, but you can decide not to be reduced by them."

~Maya Angelou

Going gluten free for Celiac disease and NCGS so you may feel reprieve from the onslaught of symptoms and stop their progression is a necessity. Living free of gluten isn't a sentence of deprivation. As you replace 'modern' SAD gluten you will naturally be introducing more real food. While stopping the destruction of your digestion and immunity while improving blood sugar regulation, your nutritional uptake is likely to soar.

If you don't currently pay much attention to your food, other than choosing food in your lane of comfort and familiarity; and eating because you need to (out of hunger/necessity, boredom, routine, etc.) you are in for a treat. You need not become a connoisseur or foodie, but since eating is the means of nourishing you for life you can begin to feel the power of choices to serve you well.

Finding joyous satisfaction from real food is a journey. It need not be an arduous journey though. You are kick starting 'freedom' as you break habits which aren't serving you well. This is freedom from food that may be perpetuating ill feelings. While you may associate restriction from food you are accustomed to eating with your journey to better living, your independence from zapped energy and symptoms reflecting a distressed body will give rise to your well-being.

Your taste will reset as your body gives up addictive qualities of the unreal food you've been eating. The mind experiences the freedom the body is feeling too. Low feelings through the process (think of stopping eating unreal food with addictive qualities as detoxing), can be very short lived. Temporary lows will lead to sustained highs as your body and mind recover from food that has been stressing you out. In return, you will feel and look more lively and energetic.

Don't underestimate the magnitude of food choices for your life. Food is a powerful force toward health or lack thereof. Food choices become very habitual and routine. While you can find wellness in routines, when habits are not serving you, it is common to be stuck in the rut of the same old food (and drink) creating more burdens in your body. Making transformative change like giving up gluten or what is not serving you well changes your experience with food for the better. You can begin to see food in a fresh way and realize it for the amazing gift it is.

The term 'gluten free' implies an association to replace food dominated by modern overly refined and processed ingredients with 'wheat' near the top of the ingredient list. Reading this book, now you know why 'gluten free' replacements can make you feel worse. They have higher sugar, unhealthy and poor quality fats, derivatives and chemicals replacing the structure gluten provides. And 'gluten free' replacements of the wheat dominant products are expensive.

Rather than choosing expensive 'gluten free' replacements (that your body loves less) consider your new food life as one *Free of Gluten*. It's a slight adjustment of thinking but a complete '180' from the overly refined ingredients and their products dominating the American food supply. Always gravitate to choose real food instead. When you lean in to packaged food, become savvy to recognize the products with minimal ingredients and those you recognize as real food. The food you want is provided by nature rather than laboratories. Your body knows what to do with real food.

You are meant for wellness. When you make this big move to eat food that satisfies you at a nourishing cellular level and soulfully, you can live the happy lifestyle you are worthy of. Ingredients are the key to a happy life. Any ingredient that doesn't serve you whether it is thought, food, drink or too much work and stress can be tuned up for improvement. Wellness is a practice. Practice is comprised of healthy habits done consistently.

You hold the powerful key to the wellness you desire with your habits. Like the saying, 'slow and steady wins the race', you can apply the same principles to replacing what does not serve you with ingredients that truly satisfy. Of course, always follow the advice of your Physician when making necessary changes. The idea is to prioritize and engage one thing at a time for longevity.

There has never been a better time to live free of gluten. New sources, recipes and labels are popping up all the time to suit a gluten restriction. When you live outside an urban area you may want for local availability of products. Some manufacturers and online retailers will ship their product to you. Sourcing on the internet, reading ingredient labels and confirming questions with manufacturers, farmers and producers will support your choices.

Keep your choices easy as possible in the beginning of your life free of gluten. Focus on easy recipes made with real food to help you shift to a new normal. Chapter 11 will delve into choosing real food. You'll find more tips to reach your new normal in Chapters 12 and 13.

In the beginning of your journey sans the gluten, you may find reprieve from eliminating gluten containing processed foods by adding in small servings (at meal times) of potatoes, other root crops/vegetables and whole grains (without gluten) like brown rice. The mentioned foods have high natural sugar content (or quickly convert to blood glucose). This is commonly referred to as the glycemic index (of a food choice) or glycemic load (referring to the meal's total impact to blood sugar).

The naturally higher 'glycemic effect' of the aforementioned foods may soothe 'withdrawal symptoms' from gluten containing processed foods. With this 'substitution', you will be getting more real food nutrition than a SAD and processed gluten diet offers. As you become more at ease without gluten containing foods, pare down higher glycemic foods to assist stable blood sugar regulation and longer burning energy. Be sure to keep quality protein and healthy fat incorporated into all of your meals and snacks to aid blood sugar regulation and energy production.

Replace wheat pasta and bread or other high carb foods (like white potatoes) with zucchini noodles (zoodles); shredded cabbage lightly steamed or sautéed; spinach; stir fried, sautéed or steamed broccoli; mashed cauliflower or cauliflower rice. Eggplant will also make a good substitution. All of these serve nicely as a bed for protein and more veggies. These foods offer higher nutrient density and won't spike blood sugar as much as wheat pasta, bread or other higher carb foods like white potatoes with a higher 'glycemic effect'. With good meal time habits like properly chewing your food, these foods are more easily digested and may ease the digestive issues you've been having with gluten or other annoying food.

Ketogenic (keto) recipes naturally don't contain high carbohydrate (SAD, wheat etc) loads making them good inspiration for a plan to eat food free of gluten. Keto choices energize you with long burning energy with emphasis on significant fat and protein content. A keto diet could be as high as 80% fat. For those coming off a high processed gluten diet, the keto plan may be distressful for digestion because an excellent ability to digest and assimilate fat and protein is needed.

Go ahead and use inspiration like that provided by Emmerich (2017). She offers recipes for 'healthified' refried 'beans' made with eggplant or zucchini. You need not focus on keto. Enjoy replacing processed wheat products with lots of real lively food.

Replace Gluten Flours

Packaged products we are accustomed to with gluten (usually labeled with wheat flour) are the foundation of cookies, cakes, bars, donuts, crackers, etc. Many of the equivalents labeled 'gluten free' often replace the gluten/wheat flour with unhealthy fats and sugar to make up for the structure gluten provides. Don't let yourself be fooled. Even when commercially baked gluten free goods are done 'in house' they can be full of extra sugar and other unwanted ingredients to replace the gluten structure.

Great alternatives serving as wonderful replacements for the 'wheat flour' dominating SAD products are homemade. Invest an hour and make a batch to realize improved nutritive value and satiation sans the gluten and other junkie food ingredients. You control all of the ingredients (aluminum free baking powder, pastured eggs, honey or maple syrup as a sweetener, sea salt, etc.) and get a more wholesome result. They usually have five to seven ingredients, all of which you can recognize as real food.

Homemade gluten free and 'paleo' cookies, bars, muffins, and cakes offer the body a much more favorable result than modern wheat flours. Not only are you foregoing the after effect of the highly refined glutinous grains, but you will support blood sugar stability. You will be satisfied longer without the chemical laden products abundant with artificial ingredients.

Double the batch without doubling your time and freeze some for another time. Because your homemade treats will be made without preservative laden ingredients, be sure to store them (and the flours) in air tight containers in the refrigerator.

Following are six of my personal favorite naturally gluten free flour products. Beyond baking, these flours are great staples for main dish cooking as breading and thickeners, all free of gluten.

Other flours not discussed here include Chickpea, Hazelnut, Oat (certified gluten free), Teff, Buckwheat, Sorghum and even Cricket flour. I haven't had experience with all of these to a great extent, but I can speak about my experience with the following alternatives to gluten containing flours. A note about Oat flour: Oats are more difficult for most people to digest, so maybe holding off on oat flour for later is a good idea if your digestion is sensitive or not up to par.

Almond flour works as a great replacement for breading, as a coating for protein; or to add to a meat loaf or meat balls as filler. It's a good replacement for a 'graham' crust. Almond flour is a good source of vitamins and minerals; is low in carbohydrates with good protein and fiber. The slightly higher protein and fat content (compared to coconut 'flour') is supportive of a low carbohydrate, ketogenic diet.   It works for baking in cookie, bar and cake recipes.   Same as with other non-gluten and grain free flours, almond flour doesn't rise.

Amaranth flour is made from ground amaranth seeds.   It has a nutty, earthy, grassy flavor that tends to take on the flavor of the ingredients it is combined with. Its protein richness is from the amino acids lysine and methionine. It is also said to be abundant in vitamins A, C and E; iron, fiber and fatty acids. Using up to 25% of amaranth flour in combination with other grain free flours like rice and coconut flour makes it a good replacement for gluten based flour when baking. It is a good thickener and breading ingredient by itself.

Coconut flour is a popular alternative to grain and gluten flours for paleo foodies and others. Made of the white meat of the inner coconut, it is highly digestible and low on the glycemic index. It is higher in fiber than almond flour with fewer calories than almond flour. Coconut flour is a good source of protein and fat. The healthy saturated fat coconut flour offers is supportive of stable blood sugar.   The Monounsaturated Fatty Acids (MUFA) make it low in Omega 6s which most people get plenty of and therefore benefit from fewer Omega 6s to balance with Omega 3s.   Coconut flour has a milder taste than almond flour.   Because coconut flour doesn't rise you will want to use it in recipes with ingredients that rise.   In addition to baked goods, pancakes, and waffles; coconut flour works well to thicken soups or stews and replaces breadcrumbs in coatings.

Cassava flour (also referred to as Manioc, Tapioca or Yuca) is derived from a tropical tuber of a shrub. It offers a sweet flavor as do many root vegetables. Tapioca pearls have been used to make pudding in this country for many years. The plant has come into recent favor by the popular culture as a 'go to' gluten free, grain free flour. It can be used as a replacement (one for one) for wheat flour and offers a mild taste and texture similar to wheat flour. The dense texture makes it appealing for cakes, cookies, brownies, tempura batter and the like.   Cassava can also be used in place of wheat or white flour as a thickener in sauces or binder in meat loafs and burger patties. When a recipe doesn't require rising, cassava flour can entirely replace the original flour. It is considered highly digestible and is a nut free alternative to almond flour. Cassava is more of the whole food from the plant, whereas tapioca is refined starch of the root. Tapioca is used to thicken sweeter sauces and make puddings. Cassava is almost pure carbohydrates with little protein or fat.

Sprouted flour is made from soaking the grain for usually 12 – 48 hours. This is a traditional method of preparing grain for consumption that removes the phytic acid. If you see reference to nutrients like B vitamins on grain products that aren't sprouted keep in mind that those nutrients are probably not going to be bio-available because the phytic acid binds them to minerals, making them more difficult for some and unavailable for others to absorb. Yellow or blue corn sprouted flour would be gluten free. Always choose organic to assure the corn wasn't genetically modified or treated with glyphosate.

Rice flour is found in many gluten free recipes. Unless it is ground superfine it tends to be grainy. A combination of superfine brown and white rice with tapioca flour and potato starch makes a good gluten free pie crust. The regular ground (not superfine) is good for breading because it is grainy. It tends to be very digestible. When you aren't going to give up pasta, choose organic brown rice pasta for a good result. Choose organic because arsenic is being found in rice crops.

Replace the Structure Gluten Provides

Acacia or Arabic Gum is from the bark of the Acacia tree and used as an emulsifier or thickener.

Agar is derived from red algae or seaweed. It is often used in place of gelatin. It is fiber rich and can help you feel satisfied longer.

Arrowroot is derived from rhizomes of tropical plants. It works well as a thickener and is often used as a replacement for cornstarch or used as a flour. Two teaspoons of arrowroot is often recommended to replace one tablespoon of cornstarch. Arrowroot forms a gel-like consistency when combined with water, making it useful for pudding, jelly/jam, cake and some sauces. It is easily digested.

Carrageenan is derived from seaweed. It is GRAS. The FDA has identified potential safety issues but it remains allowed in food.

(https://www.fda.gov/Food/IngredientsPackagingLabeling/GRAS/SCOGS/ucm261246.htm)

Guar Gum is derived from an actual food: the guar bean, or Indian cluster bean, which grows primarily in India and Pakistan. (https://chriskresser.com/harmful-or-harmless-guar-gum-locust-bean-gum-and-more/) Extensive studies have been done to evaluate potential health issues resulting from ingesting guar gum including blood glucose, cholesterol and whether it is a carcinogen. According to Kresser it makes sense to eliminate guar gum if you have sensitive digestion or any 'gut issues' (he cites SIBO and IBS). Guar gum is seen frequently in coconut milk and creamer products. It's easy to replace these products with 'guar gum' free versions.

Locust Bean Gum, or **carob gum** comes from the seeds of the carob tree. It has been used for its thickening properties, often used as an alternative for corn or wheat.

Tapioca Starch mentioned with cassava flour is a good thickener for sauces, soups and puddings. Tapioca pearls are used to make tapioca pudding. Use it in baked goods made without gluten grains. I put it in my 'Scrumptious Almond Coconut Creamer'. You can get the recipe by visiting my web page https://www.TamJohn.com. (Contact Me if you don't see the recipe)

Xantham Gum is common in gluten free baked goods because of the texture and elasticity it offers the dough. It is made from a bacterial process of a strain called Xanthomonas Campestris. The final product is considered indigestible. Lots of scientific studies have been done to know about its safety and side effects. Chris Kresser provides details on some of the studies and offers his recommendation "that people with digestive problems generally avoid xanthan gum, not because there's evidence that it could damage your gut, but because its structural properties make it likely to produce unpleasant gut symptoms." (https://chriskresser.com/harmful-or-harmless-xanthan-gum/)

Find Your New Normal

Most of us spend much of our lives away from home. There are business lunches and dinners with business associates and friends. We travel for vacation, business and weekend getaways. These are pleasures of modern life we deserve to enjoy. Eating food free of gluten or with other dietary restrictions doesn't mean you can't enjoy your on the go lifestyle.

You can adapt and learn how to choose real food wisely day in and day out without missing a beat of your life. With the following tips it becomes easy and second nature to easily and gracefully navigate life free of gluten beyond your home domain.

Restaurants

Dining out can be a great joy. Rather than relying on restaurants as a regular routine, and avoiding your kitchen, make restaurants a place to treat yourself very well. Restaurants are the locale for many a celebration, nailing down important business agendas, intimate meetings and getting food to satisfy your hunger away from home. Here you can experience foods you wouldn't normally eat. You can experience wonderful food being delivered to your table while you enjoy the company at your table while changing up your routine.

Unless you are dining in a farm to table or other unique establishment, the food on your restaurant plate is probably loaded with unreal food. The downside of a vast majority of food served to us in restaurant chains is that it has been highly processed, shaped and molded to fit the restaurant brand for consistency.

Presentation of the plated product sells. You don't see the meal slide out from its shrink wrap or as a powder before liquid is added to create sauces and sides. Overworked fryers are left with rancid vegetable oils day after day and month after month. With a little extra consideration of your restaurant choice and your menu selection, you can make restaurant dining work healthfully for you.

When dining out, your best interest is served when you thoughtfully choose the restaurant and make your menu selection. Considerations should include a restaurant venue suitable to the occasion, as well as for enjoyment and well-being. The availability of options free of gluten is offered in a wide breadth of restaurants, from casual to the finest of dining. The least likely restaurant to offer choices free of gluten is the fast food variety where you can drive through and get your food from a window if you wish.

Check out this useful site for a free of gluten dining guide in most states: http://celiac-disease.com/gluten-free-restaurants/

Some regional areas have their own free of gluten restaurant resource guides on line. Simple internet searches will turn up a variety of resources for the vast majority of locales.

Planning ahead is ideal, but when you are in a spur of the moment situation, online searches reveal restaurants exclusively free of gluten and those offering gluten free menus. Exclusively free of gluten/gluten free restaurants may give greater assurance that gluten cross contamination is null (inquire with the restaurant).

More tips to navigate healthy restaurant choices & menu selections:

❖ Most restaurants have their menu on line which allows you to review the options ahead of time.

❖ Reviewing ahead of time enables you to know there will be something you want to eat. And you can pre-think questions to ask about selections of interest to you.

❖ Even with gluten free menus, if you are Celiac or NCGS, letting the server know you are ordering gluten free due to a health necessity (you may refer to it as an 'allergy') will convey the importance and let them know gluten free isn't only a preference. So many people are 'doing gluten free' because they think it is extra healthy or in vogue without having true gluten free needs. Sometimes servers perceive the request as frivolous.

❖ Mindfully communicating with your server and restaurant staff on your very own behalf the importance of gluten free requests should get a note to the chef on your behalf.

❖ Many restaurants will cater to gluten free requests by broiling or grilling fish or other meat to avoid breading and coatings and removing sauces, etc. Striking up a rapport with your server is a great way to get the dialogue going about options.

❖ Skip the fastest food. Drive through burger joints aren't set up to accommodate gluten free diets. Save your burger craving for home when you can choose the best grass fed meat and make your burgers free of gluten.

❖ Ask if your desired meal is made in house or packaged. It may be more difficult to identify gluten free status of packaged foods.

❖ Be polite explaining your needs and asking questions. Tip generously for the extra care and consideration your server is giving you.

Ideas to modify standard gluten containing restaurant fare to be free of gluten (always confirm the details):

❖ Hamburger on a salad or bed of greens. Confirm the burger ingredients, dressings and sauces or other additions are gluten free. Beef and veggies are a great digestive combo!

❖ Naked Sandwich (without the bread) on a salad or bed of greens.

❖ Grilled fish with veggies. Skip sauces etc. likely to contain gluten.

❖ Steak and veggies. Steak and veggies are a great combination because they digest very well together.

❖ Replace pasta with broccoli, sautéed cabbage or other veggies.

❖ Sushi. Opt for sashimi and use tamari (gluten free soy sauce) or bring coconut aminos. Some sushi restaurants add sugar and flour to the rice.

❖ Taco bar. Choose toppings over salad fixings.

Gluten cross contamination may occur when gluten free foods are prepared in close proximity to gluten containing foods. Extra care must be taken in restaurants where cross contamination is likely and you don't have the control you have at home. Cross contamination may occur via toasters, colanders, cutting boards, meat slicers, sifters, double dipped utensils, fryers and storage containers, etc. Gluten containing flour may stay airborne leading to cross contamination.

Tips to confirm your food will be free of gluten cross contamination:

❖ Politely ask about preparation methods and explain your concern. Restaurants marketing 'gluten free' status will be well aware of cross contamination concerns.

❖ Ask if gluten free cooking is done in a dedicated gluten free area.

❖ Ask if your salad will be made in the same bowl as the one they use for a crouton filled salad.

❖ Ask any questions that come to mind. Your intuition will serve you well.

❖ When in doubt make another choice.

Common foods that may have gluten containing ingredients: Sauces, Dressings, Marinades, Breading/Crusts, Seasonings and Broth

❖ Ask if these items can be left off your meal or a substitute confirmed free of gluten is available.

❖ Confirm your meal when it arrives is as you ordered it.

More examples of items to be cautious about when dining out (not meant to be all inclusive):

❖ Eggs served in restaurants may have gluten containing flour batter.

❖ Some cheesecake filling is made with wheat.

❖ Burgers or meatloaf may have gluten containing fillers.

While it may seem overwhelming to ask so many questions with so much possibility for cross contamination or other inclusion of gluten in your meal, with practice of time it gets easier. You can come to know the gluten free restaurants you can rely on and menu items easiest to confirm gluten free status. Never hesitate to ask questions for clarification though. One inadvertent slip can make you feel sick for days when you are Celiac or NCGS. Communication will assure you aren't wrongly assuming anyone has your back and risk getting sick. The most important action is that you care for yourself in a way that matters for your wellness.

Travel

When communication is a barrier such as when traveling to a foreign country, using a card such as the one provided at the following link (http://www.celiactravel.com/cards/) can bridge the communication gap to add assurance your needs are understood. The server can provide this card to the chef. If they still don't understand or seem able to accommodate your needs politely go to another eatery.

When traveling anywhere, have snacks free of gluten with you. The snack list in this chapter is a good start. Avocados are also a great travel food. If you can't pack a paring knife due to air travel, you can get through the skin with a plastic knife at a fast food restaurant in the airport. Bring green unripe avocado(s) for later in your trip (time to ripen) and a ripe avocado for the first leg of the trip.

Hay, Khadro, & Dane (2014) recommend a 'Quinoa, Broccoli, and Leek Pilaf' salad for long day trips or air travel. This salad is a beauty because 'you don't have to warm it up to enjoy it', it is delicious and nutritious. The recipe is a simple combination of cooked quinoa, ghee, leek, broccoli, and seasoning. The authors offer serving and transport suggestions for travel which are applicable to other dishes you may travel with. A salad like this is an excellent example of caring for you by preparing a simple quick recipe ahead of time.

Bringing a few easy provisions on your next trip can provide a satisfying mini meal to fend off blood sugar dips and hunger pangs. Don't risk your health with the unreal food that airports or a travel situation is notorious for. Getting in a personalized wellness groove with habits to create health over your lifetime is the basis for optimal living. Make the 'on again off again' cycle of eating right and eating wrong irrelevant.

Events

Eating ahead of arriving at catered events and other gatherings will take the edge off hunger and your need to eat while supporting you healthfully. Think and plan ahead so you won't be as tempted to make a choice that will make you sick and throw you off course. I've heard people say (when they know gluten is an issue for them); they ate the cake because it was someone's birthday. Eating conventional flour cake or something else (probably commercially made) not good for you at a party because it is someone's celebration is nonsense when your body doesn't tolerate gluten. Saying 'No Thank You' is always an option. Think ahead and love yourself more!

When you are faced with tables of food at a gathering, choose the food you recognize as real. Lean in to the veggies and meats. Choose a salad with olive oil as the dressing. Upping satisfaction means choosing foods with fiber (veggies and whole fruit), and meats with protein and natural fat. The fiber, fat and protein will satisfy you. Then when you really want dessert (that you know doesn't have forbidden ingredients) indulge in moderation. Have a small piece, dish or slice. Savor each and every bite, paying attention to the food you are consuming. If it is a treat, then enjoy it!

When you are invited to bring a dish, choose one to gratify you and inspire others. It makes no sense to bring crappy ingredient dishes to any gathering or your office. For example, bring a luscious sour cream and yogurt dip with a plate of olives, veggies, salami and cheese cubes; or a hearty slow cooker chili or soup; or a plate of sliced summer veggies with olive oil and seasoning blend to be grilled at a summer barbecue. It will be a big relief to have a dish that you know is prepared with ingredients included in your eating plan. When you bring great food to events, you will plant a seed of wellness for others. Inspire others how delicious and satisfying eating for health can be.

Offering to bring a dish to support you or a family member is gracious. You may kindly let the host know that you or your other person is not able to eat a food item for health reasons and ask if you may bring something. If this conversation isn't suitable, eating ahead and then carefully choosing raw veggies, fruit, and meat without breading and other 'safe' options, you can get through the event easily. Politeness and graciousness go the distance in these circumstances, along with eating/planning ahead so you don't feel like you are dying of hunger and be tempted to make poor choices.

Kitchen Makeover

This section is your ultimate step by step guide to make your kitchen a lovely functional and healthy centerpiece of your home.

Perhaps reflecting the importance to nourish our bodies for strength, resilience, growth and life; the kitchen is where gatherings meet. It is in the kitchen where you launch your day and reconvene for reconnection at the end of the day. Arriving home from a busy day, people tend to head straight for the kitchen to find refreshment. Making your kitchen a haven with safe food and drink both nourishing for your body and soul cultivates nurturing care of yourself and loved ones.

Imagine entering your kitchen when it is time to get dinner together and you are equipped with the tools and ingredients to feed you and your family at a soulful level. A well apportioned kitchen can shift you to the point where without a specific plan, you can open the pantry and fridge and pull out a handful of food and create a simple delicious meal in a short amount of time. Time you will devote to make your kitchen compliant for your personalized wellness needs is well worth the input of energy and resources. The payoff far exceeds the investment you make.

Efficiency flows naturally when you endow your kitchen with supplies, tools and utensils ensconced in cleanliness. And with food – Real Food – you will be able to flow with nourishing the basis of life with basic ingredients. It need not be fancy. Eating for life is all about fueling your body in an easy way for *your* life.

My **Kitchen Cleanup Guide** is designed for the Celiac or NCGS person who must remove gluten. The same steps can be tweaked for anyone transitioning from a Standard American Diet (SAD) to a personalized food life.

When food like gluten is causing a health issue (Celiac and NCGS), prioritize to remove problematic foods and ingredients. Ditching junkie food is a natural extension of eating food free of gluten because commercial processed foods with gluten are the majority of the time, one and the same. You get a double whammy upside by freeing yourself of damaging gluten and the ills of highly processed and refined foods that have 'wheat' at the top of their ingredient list. You may experience a 'detox' type reaction when releasing the detrimental foods and ingredients. Some people will clear a reaction like this in a few days. Being mindful of this may help you understand what is happening if you feel the withdrawal of the food as an adjustment your body is making. Often times the reaction occurs when the body is releasing pent up toxins. Drinking extra water, getting extra sleep and being gentle with you should ease discomfort and encourage the release.

Kitchen Cleanup Guide

Get ready, pull your hair back and roll up your sleeves because this is going to be fun. You are going to thoroughly clean out, clean up and replace anything with gluten (usually has 'wheat' at the top of the ingredient list).

If you have people in your home that can safely eat gluten you may separate the gluten containing and items free of gluten in different storage. Take a long look at the ingredient labels. Don't let others (non-Celiac or non-NCGS) feast on junkie food even if they don't have an apparent issue with SAD gluten. As you are looking at labels and foods think about the havoc they create with blood sugar regulation, digestion, immunity and their nutrient deficiencies. This is a perfect time to ease the others in your home away from detrimental foods and offer more nutritious options. Everyone will benefit from more real food and less (ideally zero) junkie food.

You may be met with resistance, especially if you announce the 'great news' that you are taking away the food they are (probably unknowingly) addicted to. Silence is Golden. Silently replacing products with healthier versions for those who don't have a Celiac diagnosis may be a non-resistant way to help. As the commercial packaged cookies (or whatever) dwindle, you can shift to 'Paleo' varieties you make or purchase. Breakfast foods can shift to more protein and healthy fat containing items. Your household members will actually feel better just by changing their food. Changing the dynamics of meals and offering more real food, diminishes cravings for junkie food.

When negotiating with children or resistant adults, going about these changes silently promotes the success because there isn't an announcement to resist. When they comment on the different components of their meal or food available in the house, you can offer a slight 'hmmm, tastes good, feel better don't you?' (Along those lines of conversation with smiles) Depending on your household, the less you announce your desire to help them be healthy, the greater success you will experience. Chalk it up to human nature and how attached (addicted) people can be to their food.

In short order, those household members will begin to notice all kinds of changes like a happier mood and better feeling bodies. This is the time you may decide to ease in some dialogue to help them make great choices when they are eating away from home. This way when they are buying the food, they will have a solid basis to make great choices for their entire life and pass it on to future generations.

With gluten free and gluten eating children in the same household it is wise to dispose of all gluten containing treats. Kids have a way of getting into what they have been told is off limits. The benefits will do everybody in the house a world of good.

When 'wheat' is your target, it is easy to see it on the top of the ingredient list without need to keep reading. If you are like me, I only need to see my target to make my decision and move on. If you care to keep reading the label, you will see lots of unpronounceable (at least for me!) very long names and sugar (sometimes in several forms). Refer back to Chapter 6 for a guide to identify sugar, gauge how much you would consume if you eat 'that' product, and how products often contain sugar in several different ways. This can be extra reinforcement for your decision to ditch commercial gluten containing products.

Clean Up: Gluten travels. It floats in a fine gluten haze practically invisible through the kitchen. It attaches to towels and clothing as well as utensils and cookware. You can't always see it, so assume it is there until you clean everything up or exchange it for something new. Thoroughly wipe shelves, refrigerator, freezer, countertops and cupboards with a white vinegar and water solution. Let everything completely dry before refilling shelves and the refrigerator.

Everything - utensils, toasters, cutting boards, sifters and colanders, etc. - needs to be cleaned or replaced to be rid of gluten dust. If food has touched it, the tool or utensil must be sterilized or replaced to restore gluten free status. Utensils, sifters and colanders can be cleaned and sanitized in the dishwasher. The exception would be wooden utensils and cutting boards which should be separated or replaced. Gluten particles can remain in the wooden surfaces even after cleaning. Color code cutting boards for gluten or gluten free and store separately. Toss out old sponges for a fresh gluten free replacement. Regularly putting sponges in the dishwasher helps keep them sanitized.

Transition to Be Free of Gluten: For some people, using up food 'on the fence' (not great but not going to create an immediate health hazard as would a gluten containing product for someone with Celiac) while transitioning in more real food is a solid beginning. Transitioning away from food you already own rather than ditching it is a budget minded move. A gradual transition to homemade versions and healthier packaged options is also friendly to the body as long as you make the change. For some people this can ease anxiety about wasting food and help their body transition. You must make the change to real food for your health.

Donate unopened food items you are discarding. If it is junkie food, consider doing the less fortunate a favor and ditching it entirely. If you are able, consider a donation to your local food bank in food free of gluten and crappy ingredients. Food banks need fresh food. Spreading love like this will come back to you many fold.

Replace: As you are sorting through your cupboards, pantry and refrigerator, keep a list going with items to be replaced with food free of gluten. List making is a source for instant inspiration. Creating a habit of keeping grocery lists and meal ideas is a great way to be on top of what you need and not be 'stranded' without ingredients you want. This habit will get you through grocery shopping and meal planning with ease, saving both time and money. You'll have what you need to pull together easy, simple, nourishing and satisfying food to meet your wants and needs. More on list making in the Grocery Shopping section coming up next.

Grocery Shopping

Grocery store shelves are lined with just about anything and everything you can imagine. If you were able to ask your Great Grandmother to imagine the plethora of groceries at our arms reach she would say it is too good to be true. Well you know what the saying about too good to be true. If it seems so then it is! Let me explain.

From abundant produce departments, to shelves of yogurt flavored just about any way you can imagine and mixes for dinner, just add water and microwave it. Or don't add water and microwave it. Or just open the package and eat. Much of it isn't really food. It is a carefully crafted concoction of laboratory made ingredients designed to resemble food and keep you eating and eating and eating without the nourishment real food provides. While these choices may seem attractive from a time and taste perspective; the practice of eating like this isn't sustaining human health and well-being.

There is much good in the grocery store too. The good is in the form of real food. You will recognize it because it is grown and raised in nature or directly derived from plants or animals. Think fruit, vegetables, whole wheat berries, whole grain rice, beef, chicken, fish, butter, olive oil, etc.

Finding the good and not getting lost in the processed and refined 'food' aisles, sections and end caps luring us with addictive ingredients and attractive messages on product labels designed to reel the food into our cart takes some knowledge and practice. Knowing the fallacy behind label hype and temptation of convenience, you can make simple, easy, satisfying, nutritious and yummy choices free of gluten.

Because avoiding slip ups and bad falls is important, you must be food ready. A little planning and prep time goes a long way to bringing home real food your body can use to optimally nourish you.

‘Failing to plan is planning to fail’
(quote attribute varies to Benjamin Franklin and Alan Lakein)

The Power of the List: Don’t get caught in the trap of thinking you don’t have time to plan meals and make a thorough list of what you want and need from your grocery shopping trip. Unless you are going in for one forgotten ingredient, don’t go in without a list.

Planning ahead saves money, time and frustration in the form of extra trips to the store. Going to the store with a list targeted for the recipes and meals you will put together avoids unnecessary purchases. List making keeps you on track, focused on the real food plans you have made.

As powerful as the list is, it is also important to be flexible. Many a time I have tweaked my game plan because an ingredient wasn’t available or didn’t look good or I wasn’t willing to pay ‘that much’. Be flexible to change your game plan and add more great looking food appealing to you. Getting and staying with a real food life is about getting excited about what’s in your cart; and later your refrigerator and ultimately plate. Notice when you are drawn to the visual appeal of real food. This is your body’s petition to choose this food. Bodies know what they need and what will taste really good. The body’s signals of desire and salivation are biologically engrained to serve you.

Cravings are good. Naturally you desire different foods at different times in your life and with different seasons. Listening to this inner wisdom is your innate knowledge of what your body wants. The caveat is: If you think you are craving junkie food – You are wrong! Well actually if you haven’t kicked junkie food to the curb and reset your taste buds you may still be craving it. Chapter 11 touches more on the beauty of cravings and seasonal eating. In due time, your body won’t even want the unreal junkie food because your body will be healthfully balanced. Satisfying your sweet tooth with whole fruit; choosing energizing homemade wholesome versions of treats; and more real food will become your first nature. Listen to what your body is telling you.

Choosing the freshest and best looking food is fun. The sensory experience of enjoying food begins with grocery shopping. When you choose the most appealing fresh food available, your senses pop with imagination about eating and preparing delicious wholesome real food. Another beautiful thing about choosing the most appealing fresh food is that you can literally eat as much as you like without worry of over eating. The body is designed to be satiated when it is amply nourished.

Overly processed and refined food with chemical additives and sugar is food that doesn't signal your body for satiation. How the body handles food calorie for calorie is different with real wholesome food and the junkie food so common on grocery store shelves. One hundred calories of veggies has a much different result in the body than a one hundred calorie handful of anything processed and refined. Please your body (and mind) by choosing the freshest food each and every time you eat!

If you get snared in the trap of shopping without a list, you will likely end up eating less favorably (more eating the wrong foods for you = less satiation = more food consumption & less nutrition) and spending more money. Wasting resources is not only a waste of money but also detrimental to your vitality. Invest as much money as you can and care to on good, better and the best food. Stay in your budgetary comfort zone. You need not spend a fortune on food.

Contrary to what many believe, eating healthfully can save food budget dollars. The truth of this statement is apparent through and through what I've been saying in this book: When you eat real food you are more satiated. When you are satiated you won't be grazing for food and constantly snacking. Snack foods and energy drinks are expensive and spike blood sugar for more roller coaster eating. Real food will take you much farther energetically and financially than a junkie food diet. Buy the best food you can afford and keep it real fresh.

The idea you have to be perfect to be healthy is a fallacy. Like most things in life, wellness is a practice. Healthy habits are fortified with consistency of practice. Make small changes consistently to improve your life. Focus on real food ingredients to make nourishing yourself simple and satisfying.

Previewing weekly grocery sale flyer advertisements is a great way to prepare your game plan for meals, make your shopping list and optimize your food budget. Grocery sale ads are a great tool to plan purchases you will be stocking the pantry with. Sale ads also guide you to time a favorite recipe when its main ingredients are on sale.

Tips for planning and list making with the aid of your weekly grocery ad flyer: In a total of 20-30 minutes you will be able to review the grocery ads, while putting items on your list and jotting down meal ideas.

❖ Think of something to make on the weekend that makes great leftovers.

❖ Think seasonally. Grilling in the summer; slow cooker stew or soup in the cooler months; main dish salads in the spring, etc.

❖ Know what you are having for breakfast. List breakfast ingredients. Having a breakfast routine is a smart strategy to get your day going smoothly. You'll be able to launch your day with long burning energy when breakfast is pre-determined. (See breakfast ideas at the end of this chapter).

❖ Choose four or more fresh veggies to carry you through the week. Choose what you will eat (without spoilage) and work up to two cups of veggies in your daily food life. If two cups sounds outrageous, begin with a bite or two at one meal, then increase to each meal, working your way up to a couple of cups of veggies daily. Be sure to include leafy greens in some form. Make one of the veggies something preferred raw (carrot sticks, celery, baby greens, etc.). This way you are veggie ready straight from the refrigerator. Wash veggies (they will last longer) when you get home so they are ready to eat, steam, sauté or roast. Increasing veggies to three and four cups or even more is great news for your body when you are digesting well.

❖ Select enough fresh fruit for your household members to have a piece daily. Those with stable blood sugar regulation will be able to eat more fruit. Eat the equivalent of a cup of fresh fruit daily.

❖ Check and replenish your supply of snack food/travel/office ready food.

❖ Whatever your weakness or need, build that to strength. Whichever meal is your biggest challenge fortify your plan.

❖ Have a couple of weeknight dinners in mind with ingredients ready to go (not frozen).

❖ Have your lunch routine figured out whether it is leftovers or quick salad fixing ingredients.

'Up level' family favorites. Preferred family favorites are a good choice to stick with. You may need to 'healthify' the recipe. Change it up to incorporate quality real food ingredients to turn up your nutrition and avoid distressful ingredients like gluten. For example, if your family likes meatloaf and you are now catering to life free of gluten, make your favorite recipe and switch the gluten ingredients like bread crumbs to almond flour or quinoa.

If you've been accustomed to putting bread on the dinner table, add more vegetables or a modest serving (1/4 – 1/2 cup) whole grain rice instead of bread. Make the addition of bread special with a homemade variety.

Easy Idea: If your people like chili dogs, change the product choice to a grass fed nitrate free organic choice and gluten free chili. Forget the bun and plug in a simple veggie. Cauliflower is a nutrient dense substitute for potatoes. It is good mashed or in a side dish or soup with bacon bits. Bacon accentuates the resemblance to potatoes. Add a spoonful of raw sauerkraut as an extra goodie. Top it with a sprinkle of cheese. The result is happy and satisfied, not to mention simple, easy and delicious. This isn't a recommendation of a diet of chili dogs. The idea is to cater to your likes and make eating right easy and simple.

Over time you will find it easier to be food ready and pull together fast nutritious meals. When you are comfortable with your grocery store, you may get a rhythm of surveying sale items from the end of the aisle without walking up and down each aisle. Temptation and time are saved.

The most reliable method to choose what you will eat this week is to focus on fresh food and build a couple of meal ideas. They need not even be recipes. You can always count on a meal out of something fresh (veggies), quality protein (eggs, beef, poultry, fish) and healthy fat (real butter, olive oil, coconut oil). Veggies (something fresh and seasonal) can be sautéed in coconut oil (healthy fat) and served with a baked or grilled chicken or other meat (quality protein) in 30 minutes.

More Plan-Ahead Ideas

Plan at least one dish to be prepared on a day you are at home. Prepare something to feed you tonight and a couple more meals ahead. Soup and stew are excellent choices for the cooler months. Soup and stew are the perfect fast food and excellent for breakfast or any meal. Prepare them in a slow cooker for ease. In summer, choose grilling extra chicken or other meat for future meals. It is usually easy to make extra and doesn't double your time. Freezing some prepared items keeps you food ready.

Make a salad that is a good keeper. Check out the kale salad recipe offered in Chapter 13. The recipe is versatile for every season and preference. Kale salad will be good for at least a few days.

Make a frittata which can be breakfast, lunch or dinner. Call it 'breakfast pizza' with the kids and you'll win the little ones to the table.

If your kiddos ask if that's broccoli, inform them it is 'Brain Occoli' and pronounce it works on muscles too. Even kids want a healthy brain and strong muscles! You can have fun creating your own words for veggies and other real food. Once eaten nutrient void foods won't stand a chance in your household.

List Making Tools: Grocery list making has come a long way forward with the technology tools of our devices. Rather than carry a paper list, consider keeping your list on a device. Use your devices to track meal ideas, food journals, and recipes. Apps will help you with healthy meal and grocery planning and finding recipes. Some apps will coordinate with your calendar if that is a feature you like. A good app to meet your needs will make your life much easier and healthier. Do app store searches and check on line reviews to choose the tools which will work best for you.

Choosing the freshest most seasonal and affordable food is all about improvising. Using an iPad or other device provides a great flexibility tool for grocery shopping. For instance, I see a bunch of great looking mustard greens (or whatever) and am inspired to put them in my basket even though I don't know a thing about preparing mustard greens. I didn't know I was going to see this great looking food so it isn't on my list, but there it is, all beautiful and fresh! I am inspired to try a fresh new food I know must be healthy because it glows with vibrancy. With my iPad, I quickly scan recipes and be sure I've got the ingredients when I get home.

I keep on line recipes bookmarked on my iPad to keep my favorites close by. I won't give up my cookbook library and recipe cards with family favorites, but devices can stand up for us as a log of our wants, needs and preferences. iPads stand up nicely on the kitchen counter, for you to reference, while you are preparing the recipe.

Navigating the grocery store: Perimeter grocery shopping isn't a new idea. The problem I have with promotion of perimeter shopping is when it is promoted as if everything on the perimeter is ok and there isn't anything 'real' on the inside. Use perimeter shopping as a guideline. Long gone is the notion that you should only buy food on the perimeter. Navigate the grocery stores beginning with the perimeter. Then scan the aisles for other food you are looking for. Having a good list is your anchor to optimize your time and avoid the distraction of going through each aisle.

Grocery stores are constantly making room for new items and trying out different ideas for selling their products. Grocery stores are in the business of selling products. Buyer be aware of their methods. There is nothing wrong with selling food. People need food. But much of the marketing and methods of the grocery business has grown beyond the best interests of food eating people. Grocers are clever about interspersing less than ideal and very profitable items on the perimeter and at eye level. For instance, all yogurt isn't 'created equal' and this applies for every product category in the store. Thinking that yogurt is healthy because it is on the perimeter, isn't absolute. Become familiar with labels and brands that serve what your body needs. Check back with the label to be sure the ingredients haven't changed.

Buying groceries takes the mindset of a persistent sleuth to keep what you put in your body on a healthy course. I recently stopped at one of my favorite grocery stores to pick up a sale item that they had run out of on my regular trip. My plan was to go in for that item only. I was thirsty though, and although I had water I wanted something more flavorful. I stopped at the beverage cooler with the bottled teas. I was expecting some sugar, but when I started reading beyond the 'natural and slightly sweet claims' I found as much as 36 grams of sugar in one bottle. Thirty six grams is over seven teaspoons of sugar in a 12 ounce bottle claiming it 'natural' (implying healthful). Do yourself a favor and always check a label for ingredients and facts like grams of sugar. Be sure to look at the serving size too, since the label may indicate multiple servings in a bottle.

The most profitable grocery items for sale are placed where you are most likely to see them and put them in your cart. Being aware of this, visually scan the bottom shelf when there is a product in the category you are looking for. You may find a 'cleaner' version at a lesser price than eye level shopping. For example, I prefer plain organic green tea (no fruity or tropical varieties or blends). My preferred 'clean' organic plain green tea is presumably on the bottom shelf because it is the least expensive. Green tea is loaded with antioxidants and is said to promote heart health, healthy blood pressure and blood sugar, and be good for bones and vision. It is smack in the middle of the store, along with many other real food items including nuts and seeds and useful staple items like almond flour and rice. Canned wild salmon, tuna and sardines are in the middle of the store. Some brands of these items are very healthful and lively. You'll also find olive oil, olives and coconut oil in the middle of the store, along with many other quality real foods.

Being a savvy shopper and avoiding unwanted ingredients like SAD gluten isn't about staying only in the perimeter. Being a savvy shopper is about knowing labels, identifying real food ingredients and first and foremost choosing real fresh lively food as a priority.

When meals are comprised of the freshest food, usually found on the perimeter (think produce, meats, butter, eggs, etc.) you are eating optimally for health, energy, growth and restoration.

Going in, with your game plan and list;   here's your step by step to navigate the grocery store with savvy skill:

1. Take Cooler Bags. Keep your food at the right temperature until you can properly refrigerate, freeze and store at home.

2. Select Fresh Foods First. Your body thrives on fresh food. It is the best source for a variety of nutrients. Stay focused on buying fresh food to alleviate the issue of evaluating ingredient labels because with real food, there isn't an ingredient label. The food IS the ingredient. Satisfy your list with the best fresh food the store has available today. Choosing fresh foods first builds the center of your eating plan. Select what you know you can eat while it is still fresh or you are able to freeze or otherwise preserve. Many items like meat, eggs and dairy are dated. You will find dates on packaged produce items like greens. Most produce items should be eaten within five days.

Organically grown and raised fresh food doesn't present a chemical burden for your body. If you can't afford to buy everything organically grown, prioritize organic purchases. Choose organic produce items with skin that gets consumed (i.e. apples and berries). Items like bananas and avocados which you don't consume the skin isn't as high priority to choose organic. The Environmental Working Group (ewg.org) publishes *THE EWG's 2017 GUIDE TO PESTICIDES IN SHOPPER'S PRODUCE* ™ named the *Dirty Dozen*™ and *Clean Fifteen*™ as guides to assist prioritizing organic purchases. The EWG lists sweet corn on the *Clean Fifteen*™ list. In my opinion sweet corn must be organic to avoid ingesting chemicals. Perhaps it is the husk which keeps it protected from chemicals; however, corn is a primarily genetically modified and sprayed crop in the United States.

Be sure to wash produce which will aid removal of unwanted substances and dirt and keep it fresher longer. Use a white vinegar and cool water solution, about 1 part vinegar: 5 parts water. Salt water works nicely to clean cruciferous veggies. Rinse well, dry (or spin dry greens) before storage.

Buy fresh food grown and raised close to home when possible. The closer it is picked, grown or raised to home should mean a higher nutritional value. Distantly grown food is picked prior to being ripe, putting a damper on its nutritional value. Produce tags usually will tell you the locale the item originated from.

Beyond produce, fresh foods include wild fish in season (preferably not frozen first), locally raised grass fed and pastured meats, pastured and organic eggs, and grass fed butter. Other artisan type items may be available in your area like kombucha and other fermented foods, cheeses and bread (not the commercial bakery ingredients, but real artisan items). Some artisan breads are made without gluten containing grains or are made with organic and traditional methods like sourdough or sprouted grains. Prepared and semi-prepared items made with real food ingredients can make it easier to bring real good food into busy schedules.

3. Avoid prepackaged gluten free items like cookies, crackers and other baked goods. The gluten is often replaced with lots of sugar, manmade chemicals, preservatives and additives the body wasn't designed to assimilate. It's easy to find recipes to make gluten free 'Paleo' cookies, bars, pancakes, crackers and other items. Making crackers from nut milk pulp is easy, delicious and satisfying. These crackers don't contain flour. The protein punch you get from the nut crackers gives you a big wallop of satisfaction for long burning energy you won't get from grain based flour crackers. There are some decent free of gluten, minimal ingredient and real food ingredient crackers and cookies on grocery shelves today. Cover your bases by reading labels. Then choose to eat prepackaged items occasionally rather than as a staple.

Homemade nut milk is so much better tasting and free of chemicals than the store bought variety. When you make a homemade batch of anything, you will know exactly what goes in your food. You will experience feeling fuller sooner, eat less and receive more nutritive value. Going homemade is a lot less expensive and much more delicious than prepackaged items too. Find a window of time to make an item here or batch there. The result to your food life is reshaped deliciously and nutritiously. Take action to remove what ails you and gravitate toward more real food.

Gluten can show up just about anywhere in packaged food products (refer to Chapter 3). Reading labels diligently and looking for gluten free labeling and certification (refer to Chapter 5) will save you time when you think you must choose a packaged product. Even the most seemingly inoffensive product may have unwanted ingredients. Nuts, as an example, often contain coatings, sugar and preservatives. Choose raw nuts instead of the addictively coated varieties. To support sensitive digestion raw nuts can be soaked and gently dehydrated. *Nourishing Traditions* (1999) cookbook has a wonderful recipe for

'Crispy Nuts' that follows the time honored tradition of soaking and gently dehydrating nuts to reduce phytic acid.

There are 'like for like' food options without extra unwanted ingredients for just about everything. The 'better for you' products will give you a better feeling after consumption. It will be as if you are reaping a payoff of caring for yourself in a delicious and easy manner. You feel better. Soon you can have your favorite options scoped out and be able to cruise through grocery shopping with ease. Your diligence for choosing fresh food, free of gluten or whatever doesn't agree with you, can become your first nature.

4. Stock your Pantry with Simple Basics. Having items like sweet potatoes, quinoa and brown rice on hand for side dishes is easy and inexpensive. They store well, making it easy to have them in your pantry. Transforming your food choices to please your body requires being mindful of the time investment, and keeping your food and meal plans simple.

Optimizing time, money and nutrition is a strategy that varies personally. Your needs change and evolve over time. Make choices that feel rewarding. Diminishing symptoms, weight loss without deprivation, better sleep, more relaxation and spending less money on your total food budget can become a lifestyle you love.

Healthy for You Food Ready Hacks

❖ Make pesto from greens like arugula, basil, cilantro, spinach and root veggie tops (carrots & beets). Mix and match the greens for your taste and what you've got on hand or look the liveliest at your market. Pesto is easy to make and freezes well. It is a nutritious ingredient for a quick meal to be added to rice pasta, rice or as a marinade for chicken or pork. Total time: 15 minutes.

❖ Freeze cut pineapple and clean berries in small packages for snacking, smoothies or a gluten free berry cobbler. Total time: 10 minutes.

❖ Veggies like green beans are easy to blanch (put in boiling water for 2 – 3 minutes) and seal in plastic bags for the freezer. Total time: 20 minutes

❖ Buy frozen veggies (just veggies on the ingredient label) on sale for a quick meal ingredient. Some people say frozen is optimal because it is flash frozen when picked at the peak of ripeness. Total time: one to two minutes.

❖ Make your own trail mix with your favorite nuts, seeds, dried fruit, carob or cacao and coconut chips. You'll be assured of the ingredients you want without any added sugar or preservatives. Keep them in small containers or sandwich/snack baggies so they are ready to grab and go. Total time: 30 minutes.

❖ Make a double batch of baked goods or pancakes (see my recipe in this book for pumpkin or applesauce pancakes) and freeze extra. Use wholesome ingredients your body loves. Reap the reward of more energy and satisfaction than commercial products laden with unwanted ingredients. Total time: one hour.

❖ Buy from a bulk warehouse. This is a great buying spot for organic rice, wild canned salmon, wild fresh and frozen fish, organic chicken, almond flour, coconut oil, nut butter, fruit, veggies, grass fed butter, raw sauerkraut, bone broth and many other real foods and ingredients. Total time: one hour.

❖ When you won't eat a bulk package before spoilage, freeze it in smaller portions easy to pull out for a meal in the right size. Total time: 15 – 30 minutes.

❖ Invest in a grass fed beef portion direct from the rancher. Quantities as small as 1/8 are available. You can purchase pastured lamb and pork direct from ranchers too. Some deliver to your home.

❖ Buy large packages of meat (less per pound) and freeze with a food sealing system in package sizes right for you. Label packages with contents and date. Total time: 30 minutes.

❖ Look into the new online grocery retailers. Thrive Market (http:// thrv.me/7xL45S) (referral) has become a favorite of mine. In addition to the convenience (and time savings) of having non- perishable groceries delivered to my door, I've found the prices are a great savings over the items I was buying in a brick and mortar store. Total time: 30 minutes or so (so much more saved depending on travel time).

❖ Meal ingredient delivery. There are quite a few being advertised. They portray fresh ingredients and recipes delivered to your door. Couldn't be easier!

❖ Personal Chef. This is sure to pick up momentum. Personal chefs will come to your home with all ingredients, utensils, pots, pans, etc. and prepare a menu offering you have selected of dinners for a couple weeks. The meals are refrigerated or frozen and you simply heat them.

❖ Have a 'To Go Food Pack' ready in your desk drawer (or suitcase if you are traveling) for those days when the best laid plans go awry & you didn't bring lunch, you can't go out to lunch, you have to work late, breakfast at home wasn't an option, or you have a blood sugar dip and need to stabilize. Fill your 'To Go Food Pack' with cans of wild salmon, paleo meat bars, jarred artichokes, garbanzo beans, raw nuts, pumpkin seeds, almonds, etc. Make it a weekly practice to take a couple pieces of whole fruit to the office. Have a whole lemon cut in wedges to add to your water. Include organic tea bags. Keep sparkling water and purified water at the office.

Preserve Some Food

Quality grocers will help you capitalize on opportunities to stock up for time and money savings. Watch the weekly sale ads and stock up on items suitable for you and your household. Ask your grocer for case discounts on seasonal produce if you are willing to preserve it. Seasonal peaches, apples, green beans, tomatoes and berries are commonly preserved items. Learning to do water bath or pressure canning isn't too difficult. Classes are often held through County Extension offices and other resources. Dehydrators are popular for dehydrating fruit and nuts. Demonstrations are plentiful on YouTube.

Preserving even a little bit of food will be a treat for you in the winter months. Imagine your (made in advance) homemade stew or chili thawing and slowly reheating in a slow cooker on a cold winter day and you didn't have to leave the house or do much of anything in the kitchen. Imagine thawing pesto, gently heating homemade tomato sauce or snacking on dehydrated apple slices and crispy nuts …. There are many wonderful options to preserve a little or a lot and be food ready. Discover some food preservation appealing to you. Involving a friend or child is a great way to have some old fashioned fun, create memories and maybe even a new tradition.

More Inspiration

Have fun. More time in the kitchen can be fun regardless of your cooking skills. Put on great music while you move around your ingredients and create delicious meals. Keeping meals and food prep simple with just a few ingredients will keep feelings of being overwhelmed way down.

Fun kitchen games might include 'contests' with your family or housemates to create the most color in a dish or salad; or the most delicious meal with the fewest ingredients; or the quickest healthy dinner prep. The possibilities for being a wildly fantastic cook or just a darn good creator of real simple food are endless. Relax and ease into choosing food that deeply nourishes you.

Slow Down. Taste, chew and enjoy the food you are eating. Think about how it grew and maybe even its journey to your table. Mindfulness creates gratitude. Slow down and set the stage for optimal enjoyment and digestion of your food.

Treat Yourself. Buy something you really love, and know is good for you. Maybe you love a great cut of wild fish. Buy the best darkest chocolate you can afford. Maybe your treat is a great smoothie. Invest in the best ingredients, make almond milk (it's really easy and so much better than store bought), put in the most beautiful berries and a few of the prettiest spinach or kale leaves with a dollop of pumpkin… do something so decadent and good for you that you feel pleasure when you taste it. Savor each morsel, and taste the goodness your treat offers.

Meal Planning Ideas

Your well-endowed kitchen (newly made over and well-stocked) gives you the platform to have lively food ready to go for nourishing benefits.

Nourishing satisfaction is complemented when the meal setting is calm, peaceful and pleasant. 'Ground rules' for meal time at your home may include putting devices and television aside; an attractive table; no figuring out problems or having difficult conversations; and anything else to promote a pleasant experience. A calming peaceful setting promotes optimal uptake of the nourishment you have prepared and put on your table and plate. Relax and enjoy a respite from a busy day, even if just for 20 minutes. When 20 minutes of calm is comfortable, raise the bar and enjoy yourself for 30 minutes while you savor your food and table company. When dining alone, this is your time to be completely self-focused, putting on lovely music and settling into the sensory experience of your meal.

There is no need to plan out every meal in detail or ascribe to the burden of perceived perfection to prepare a 'square meal'. Having allowable ingredients you like, and those in agreement with your body, sets the stage for ease of meal preparation. With a little pre-thought, most days you need not exceed 30 minutes to pull a meal together.

Easy meal routines are made of simple basics.

Always have at least one thing fresh or raw. Always include quality protein and healthy fat. Carbohydrates should be primarily veggies. Anything else you add is at your scrutiny of what it brings to the meal for your nourishing satisfaction. Every way you choose to approach easy meals comprised on nourishing lively food becomes a practice.

Carbohydrates should be primarily veggies. Something raw can be as easy as carrot sticks, zucchini rounds, small handful of baby greens, an apple, etc. Now in the habit of stocking your crisper drawer with washed fresh produce, this practice becomes easy. Begin answering the question 'what's for dinner' starts with your crisper drawer. Decide your method: Roasting, Steaming, Sautéing, Pureeing, etc. Use healthy cooking fat if applicable; and/or add a drizzle of healthy fat for topping.

By nature's design, quality protein is paired with healthy fat. Your choice can be as simple as canned wild salmon. It is a decent fast option for a busy person. Wild fish in season offers fast preparation, less than 10 minutes. Frozen wild fish is a good choice in the off-season. Baking chicken is an easy one dish solution for quality protein. Grass fed organic hot dogs make a decent protein option in a pinch (example in previous chapter). Grass fed ground beef can be cooked as meatloaf, burgers, taco meat (with veggies like cauliflower and peppers and onions diced and added). These quick ideas are as perfect as a quality protein component needs to be for a simple meal.

Throwback to the days when one night of the week was for one food: It went something like this: Monday night is leftover Lasagna (you can make it with eggplant or butternut squash instead of noodles); Tuesday is Taco Tuesday; Wednesday is chili dogs, Thursday is chicken and Friday is fish. Give your family what they like as a 'new and improved' version. On Saturday or whichever day you are off work, plan a great restaurant night when you can explore a new choice or visit an old favorite (with options in your food life plan). If you enjoy cooking, prepare a new recipe when you have the leisure. Over the weekend you can reset your game plan for the new week with grocery shopping and some prep while involving your household team and build to everyone's strengths.

Maybe you are the overseer and primary planner, but your husband, partner or roommate can bring in and put away groceries; someone washes veggies, someone makes this or chops that. Someone is the primary cook or dishwasher/dryer. Single dwellers can relish that all of the amazing food is for you. Choose everything you love, enjoy all the leftovers and turn the kitchen music up as loud as you care.

More Meal Ideas

* Recipe available in Chapter 14

Breakfast

❖ Scrambled eggs with baby spinach, bacon or sausage. Cook the eggs low and slow to preserve delicate nutrients.

❖ Hardboiled egg and baked sweet potato with butter and sour cream. Have eggs ready to go, even peeled, if it makes your morning routine easier. When you wake, put the sweet potato in parchment slathered in coconut oil, place in baking dish and bake for about an hour or more at 425 degrees while you get ready for your day.

❖ Leftovers of quality protein like beef, chicken, turkey or fish with veggies from last night's dinner. Quality protein like this will certainly set you up with long burning fuel for your day.

❖ Soup or stew. Why not eat leftover slow cooker soup or stew for breakfast. Sure to fuel you for the day! This might be the perfect fast food.

❖ Veggie omelet (baby spinach, diced multi-color peppers, green onion) with ½ prebaked potato or sweet potato cubed and browned to golden in coconut oil.

❖ *Pumpkin pancakes with bacon or sausage and egg (scrambled, over easy or hardboiled) with drizzle of maple syrup or honey. The pancakes can be made ahead and frozen in small packages. Thaw and reheat. Ditto for the bacon or sausages (cook ahead, and reheat).

❖ Greek style whole fat plain yogurt with drizzle of honey and sprinkle of raw nuts like almonds, walnuts or pumpkin seeds.

❖ Quinoa porridge or 100% buckwheat cereal served in warm unsweetened almond milk with quality protein like ham, sausage or egg.

Lunch

❖ Salad made at home with variety of in season veggies and 4-6 oz (about the size of your palm) of quality protein like wild fish/salmon, chicken or turkey. Think tender greens, colorful peppers, celery, carrots, radish, cucumbers, summer squash and cabbage.

❖ *Kale salads are excellent keepers to make ahead. Add protein for long burning energy.

❖ Grass fed hamburger patty served on bed of baby spinach or other greens. Top it with a slice of cheese and a bacon strip if it agrees with you. Add all the veggies you can muster.

❖ Gluten free grass fed hot dog with gluten free chili and raw veggie sticks.

❖ Almond butter on allowable grain toast, raw veggies and grass fed cottage cheese sprinkled with raw sunflower seeds.

❖ Leftovers from dinner: Quality protein and veggies.

❖ Tostada made with brown rice tortilla, black beans, ground meat (beef, chicken or turkey), green onions, avocado, tomatoes, cheese and salsa.

❖ Fish tacos or tostado made with pineapple salsa and served in organic corn or brown rice tortilla shell. Serve with black beans, wedge of lime and sliced grape or pear organic tomatoes and cucumber if in season.

Dinner (*make extra for leftovers for breakfast & lunch*)

❖ Homemade stew from the slow cooker is wonderful to come home to and makes great leftovers for any meal.

❖ Soup made in the slow cooker is a great fast food. Choose chicken, turkey, beef and lots of veggies.

❖ Roast chicken from the slow cooker with carrots, potatoes, veggies. Making bone broth from the remains is easy and nourishing.

❖ Stir fry with chicken and veggies.

❖ *Broccoli and beef over brown rice or quinoa or sautéed cabbage with tamari or coconut aminos.

❖ *Pork carnitas.

❖ *Quinoa 'fried' rice.

❖ Baked wild fish with lemon wedge, steamed green beans and baked sweet potatoes or baby red potatoes. Top with butter or olive oil.

❖ *Grilled lemon chicken & veggies.

❖ *Crispy chicken tenders & veggies sautéed in coconut oil.

Snacks

❖ Whole fruit (Just one piece of whole fruit daily if you have any blood sugar issues).

❖ Smoothie made with unsweetened almond, cashew or coconut milk, berries, with a little spinach or kale and organic hemp hearts. Add a dollop of pumpkin for extra goodness. Homemade nut milk is the best. It is easy to make.

❖ Cookies or macaroons made from nut milk pulp.

❖ Raw nuts or pumpkin seeds with dried fruit. Keep dried fruit servings small since it has high sugar content.

- Homemade snack bars made with chopped dried fruit, nut butter, little honey, gluten free grains.
- Paleo meat bars. There are many brands and varieties. Try one at a time to be sure you like it. Beef, chicken, turkey and salmon are available.
- Veggie sticks with hummus. Hummus can be made from garbanzo beans, parsnips, or beets.
- Dehydrated beet or sweet potato chips with yogurt & sour cream dip or hummus.
- Plain whole fat yogurt with a drizzle of honey & sprinkle of raw or soaked and dehydrated nuts.
- *Homemade cookies free of gluten. The amazing thing about homemade cookies free of gluten is they don't have the wheat and artificial ingredients to wreak havoc with blood sugar and digestion. Look for recipe options without refined sugar. These are very satisfying when made with high protein almond flour.
- Canned wild salmon (with a squeeze of lemon), nitrate free summer sausage, jarred olives, jarred artichoke hearts and garbanzo beans with fresh veggie slices like carrots, red/yellow/orange bell peppers, zucchini, parsnip, radish, few spinach leaves, etc. … add yogurt & sour cream homemade dip and you have a robust snack plate or meal replacement that doesn't require cooking.

More Real Food Sources

Farmer's markets to procure real food grown close to home have been in existence for many years. Farmer's markets are held in all sizes of cities, towns and communities. Sometimes they found road side or in parks and other community locations. The grower or vendor sets up a table or booth and sells their goods. The social aspect of browsing farmer's market booths and tables while mingling among people and their dogs in a casual setting can be tons of fun.

It's environmentally appealing to shop at farmer's markets because the 'footprint' to deliver food to its consumer is much more favorable than when food is grown at a long distance from its consumer. Food sold here can be picked at ripeness for the consumer which optimizes nutrition and freshness.

To reap healthy benefits of a farmer's market, be aware that produce and other items like baked goods may not meet standards for being free of gluten, organic or GMO-free.

Although many of the items sold at these markets may be very good for you, be aware of what is in it and how it was grown or raised to know what you are getting. Vendors generally encourage a dialogue with consumers about how their produce is grown or other items are made. Let the vendor know you can't ingest gluten (or whatever) for health reasons and ask about their ingredient and growing methods.

Organic certification can be very costly. While it may not be feasible for growers who participate in farmer's markets to be certified, the grower may use organic means to cultivate and grow the crops they provide. Ask them how they deal with pests and about their farming methods to guide you. This way you can be certain they are practicing your preferences.

Community Supported Agriculture (CSA) is a means for farmers and consumers to share risk and reward of farming operations. The consumer pays an annual fee to the CSA. This membership entitles the consumer to share the farm's bounty. Risk and reward is shared accordingly. If the farm has a bad season due to a weather event or other circumstances, the shareholder won't receive as much bounty. The shareholder either picks up produce or other goods weekly at the farm or a pickup location nearer the residential area of the shareholders is provided. See Resources for a CSA Directory.

Chapter 11

Up Level Your Life with Real Lively Food

"You don't have to cook fancy or complicated masterpieces, just cook food from fresh ingredients."

~Julia Child

Real food is a nourishing investment for health and vitality. Adding 'lively' to the equation [Real Lively Food] indicates the connection of real food and wellness. It is alive with nutrition which translates to fuel for your body and mind. Whether you are enjoying your wellness groove and interested in expanding it, or attending to signs and symptoms for their reversal, choose real lively food to up level your life. Your food choices impress how you live today, tomorrow and years from now.

Many Americans believe they eat 'clean and healthy' enough. In reality, the food dominating their diet includes meal replacement bars loaded with sugar and chemicals; protein shakes with adulterated ingredients and more laboratory made derivatives than real food. Overly processed food is often disguised as 'healthy' or 'natural' according to the slippery slope where modern culture meets food marketing. The price of poor choices is ill health.

Michael Pollan (2008) eloquently wrote 'You are what you eat eats...' Pollan's expressiveness is a reflection of the interconnected nature between humanity, our food supply and environment. Our beautifully designed planet began with plants (fruits and vegetables) grown and nourished in a natural environment (sunshine, rich soil and rain fall). Animals for consumption roamed and ate foods naturally beneficial for them, following their biological programming. At the advent of ranching, animals were bred and raised in settings where they could roam and eat foods their body was designed to digest for optimal well-being. Today's commercial feed lot animals are typically raised in confined and unnatural settings and fed diets comprised of foods unnatural for them to digest. Practices like this make them more susceptible to dis-ease and may cause a greater need for drugs like antibiotics. When the natural process of nourishment and life is honored, the vegetation and animal's increased vitality is evident in the food it provides us. Human nutrition works similarly. When we eat the wrong food, our function struggles to some extent. Left unattended dysfunction increases over time becoming more burdened and creating a cascade of dis-ease and dis-comfort.

You weren't designed to have food intolerances, digestive distress, insomnia, mood/attention/depressive disorders, etc. with their high prevalence in America. What you eat matters to your health and well-being, all of which contribute to longevity. According to Dr. Hyman (2016), while there are significant genetic differences in how people handle fats and carbs, we all do better on a whole foods diet. He cites the Standard American Diet as the worst diet on the planet.

Select the highest quality food you can afford as a measure for wellness. Choosing quality protein and healthy fat, with veggies as your primary carbohydrates at every meal will boost your energy and replace frequent snacking. The long lasting smooth energy you will feel can save money on your food budget when you follow this basic premise. Naturally you will forego processed snack foods, energy drinks and fancy commercial coffee drinks, all of which are expensive and largely void of any actual upside. Your desire for food largely void of an upside will vanish when you are satisfied with real lively food.

A Fresh Wellness Mindset is never about deprivation. Chapter 12 dives into how to create a food life with plenty of room to include food that tastes decadent and is intensely satisfying. Keep the triple combination of protein, fat and veggies as a food model to serve as your foundation. Balancing wellness is about modifying your food intake based on how you feel and your energetic needs.

When your digestion and blood sugar regulation are in need of restoration, focus on making the simplest food choices with intent to mend this function. When you begin to feel better and signs and symptoms of distress are diminished, it is a good time to begin introducing more complexity and richness into your food plan.

The single nutrition question I am most commonly asked is whether someone should eat a plant based diet. My answer is always yes. Please let me explain what a plant based diet means to me. My idea of a plant based diet is a lunch and dinner plate with primarily vegetables, with a serving of quality protein and a little healthy fat.

An ample serving size of quality protein for most people is about the size of their palm. Healthy fat may be a tablespoon of butter, drizzle of olive oil, or veggies sauteed in a tablespoon of coconut oil. Overboard anything may be counterproductive. As with every component of *A Fresh Wellness Mindset*, some experimentation is necessary to find what feels the best for you. At different times in your life you may need a little more or less protein and fat depending on metabolic needs.

Dr. Weston A. Price studied a vast number of indigenous diets around the world in the 1930s. He found a wide variety in the diets of healthy people. All healthy diets included some form of animal protein. In some instances it was bugs. Crickets are now in vogue, so maybe that is for you! The Dali Lama is said to eat animal protein from time to time. Finding the right source and amount of protein for your body's needs is vital for optimal wellness.

Choosing to forego animal protein in the diet requires a targeted approach to be sure food choices are covering nutritional needs. Since vitamin B12 is found in animal foods, if a person chooses to be animal protein free, supplementation with vitamin B12 is a necessity. Methylcobalamin is the active form of B12. This is the specific form of B12 needed for nervous system health. Because of methylcobalamin's importance in nervous system health, it is also an important nutrient for vision. (http://www.dadamo.com/B2blogs/blogs/index.php/2004/02/07/cyanocobalamin-versus-methylcobalamin?blog=27)

Since vitamin B12 is vitally important for cardiovascular, brain and nervous system health and DNA production, it is a good idea to ask your Physician or Naturopathic Doctor to test your level of B12. If you are supplementing, be consistent. Vitamin B12 is water-soluble (your body will not store it in fat tissue). If you need to adjust your B12 level you can easily modify your dosage to get to your ideal level.

As a guideline, most bodies will do well with about 15 – 25% of dietary caloric consumption as protein; about 30 – 60% as fat; and 25 - 50% carbohydrates, primarily veggies. Paying attention to how you feel (energy, mood, sleep, signs, symptoms or lack thereof, etc.) is the key to personalize dietary intake just right for you. Your body's need for protein, fat and carbohydrates will vary over your lifetime. Be mindful about how you feel to tap in to your body's needs and make dietary adjustments.

Veggies should make up the majority of your carbohydrates (carbs). Carbs are needed for brain fuel and a quick source of energy for muscles. Carbs work with protein and fat to regulate metabolism; fight infection, promote growth of bones and skin and lubricate joints.

Carbs provide fiber which helps eliminate toxins through the large intestine. Vegetable sources of carbs create ideal blood glucose (sugar), just as nature intended. Veggies don't turn to blood glucose as quickly as refined and processed foods so their effect on blood sugar regulation is ideal to fuel your brain and muscles. Processed and refined carbohydrates won't give you anywhere near the spectrum of nutrition you receive when you choose a diverse array of colorful vegetables.

In our modern world, virtually every vegetable is available to us year round. Fresh seasonal veggies are ideal. Fresh veggies grown hundreds and thousands of miles away from your locale are not picked at the peak of ripeness. Ripeness implies the peak of nutritional availability. I don't think anything beats a locally grown (home garden is best!) vegetable for taste, texture and nutritional zest.

Frozen vegetables can add diversity and ease depending on where you live and the season. Frozen veggies are said to be optimally nutritious because they are picked at the peak of ripeness and soon thereafter blanched and flash frozen. Check their ingredient labels since some may contain sugar or other unwanted ingredients. Frozen veggies will also state the country of origin. Stocking up on frozen vegetables on sale is a smart strategy for eating well and within a budget, especially the winter months when fresh supplies may not be as plentiful. Use them before they get freezer burn and nutrients diminish.

When you begin moving to more real foods in your eating regimen, veggies may be somewhat foreign. Keep it simple and select what you like. Carrots and baby lettuce might be a good beginning. Gently steaming carrots and other veggies (not lettuce though) can make them more palatable to someone who isn't accustomed to crunchy food.

Begin raw veggie consumption slowly. They require more digestive power. Gently cooking veggies aids their digestion by breaking down the fibrous content. Gently is the key word, since over cooking can utterly deplete the nutritional benefits and turn them to mush. Beta carotene is said to be more bio available when carrots, for example, are gently cooked. Other nutrients like vitamin C may be decreased, while the beta carotene is enhanced, so change up the cooking methods you use. Adding new veggies and veggies of different varieties and grown in different soils keeps the nutrient (especially mineral) content varied.

Try these ideas to up level your enjoyment of veggies:

❖ A little drizzle of quality extra virgin olive oil with spritz of fresh lemon and dash of sea salt or drizzle of untoasted sesame oil and sprinkle of sesame seeds may be all you need to delight your taste buds.

❖ Add a pat of butter for a savory finish.

❖ Some kids, big and small, are won over with a sprinkle of cheese added to veggies.

❖ Various methods of cooking vegetables include baking, roasting, steaming, blanching and sautéing.

❖ A simple sauté in coconut oil makes eating zucchini, onion, and peppers all diced with a little sea salt delicious.

❖ Color reflects nutrients. To preserve the full nutritional complement of vegetables, do not overcook them. Recognize the full nutrition by serving them when they are still brightly colored.

❖ Save the cooking water for a soup or broth base to preserve the nutrients for another use (or drink it).

❖ Lettuces are usually eaten raw although watercress is delightful slightly wilted.

When you are moving away from a processed diet and SAD gluten, having a real (ideally organic) potato (or sweet potato) with butter and real sour cream with dinner can sooth your withdrawal from processed food. Introducing root vegetables in place of overly processed and refined grains will support more stable blood sugar than SAD grains because they are real food without additives, preservatives, other chemicals and sugar commonly part of a grain based food product. Carrots, potatoes (white, red, yellow, purple), sweet potatoes, yams, parsnips, turnips, rutabagas, radish, celeriac and beets are all root vegetables. A baked sweet potato with a pat of butter and quality protein (nitrate free sausage, leftover chicken, fish, turkey, beef, or hardboiled egg) is a satisfying breakfast (or any meal) and supportive of healthy blood sugar regulation.

Root vegetables are known for being especially rich in vitamins A and C, potassium, magnesium and fiber. These starchy vegetables offer complex carbohydrates. They are naturally seasonally available toward the end of summer and early autumn. They are higher in sugar than other veggies making them available seasonally to promote energy storage (more fat) for ancestral man during the winter months. Their seasonal availability made them a crop American pioneers (without access to other fresh food in the winter months) relied upon. Root vegetables store well although avoid refrigeration for potatoes because the starch will convert to sugar making the sugar content as high as a candy bar.

As you are getting established as a regular veggie eater, you can lean into the many other vegetable choices to dominate your veggie consumption. Choose a colorful variety of vegetables for a diverse palate of nutrition. Spring and summer bring leafy greens, a rich source of alkalinizing minerals, vitamins C, E and K, and many B vitamins. Leafy greens have phytonutrients such as beta-carotene (the pre-cursor for vitamin A), lutein and zeaxanthin. These nutrients are said to protect cells and eyes. The darkest green vegetables contain some Omega 3s. Chlorophyll, a super anti-oxidant, is abundant in leafy greens. Choose often from the lettuces, escarole, arugula, spinach, kale, collards and mustard greens.

Cruciferous veggies are members of the Brassicaceae (also called Cruiciferae) family. They contain sulfur-containing glucosinolates which gives them a distinctive taste and is said to support detoxification. They contain Indole-3-carbinol said to be anti-cancer. Cruciferous veggies include cabbage, broccoli, kale, collard greens, cauliflower, mustard greens, Brussels sprouts and bok choy. Cruciferous veggies may be contraindicated with thyroid health in some people because they contain goitrogens which impede the uptake of iodine necessary for thyroid function.

Yellow and orange vegetables contain zeaxanthin, flavonoids, lycopene, potassium, vitamin C and beta-carotene. Like other veggies, the yellow and orange varieties are especially supportive for eyes and bone health. They are strong supporters for immune system health, promote healthy joints and collagen, lower blood pressure, fight free radicals and support prostate health. Choose winter squash including spaghetti, butternut, pumpkin, yellow summer squash, sweet potatoes, carrots, and yellow beets, orange and yellow peppers.

Purple and dark red vegetables are among the richest in anti-oxidants. The purple pigment in these vegetables contains flavonoids, including resveratrol, which can help decrease blood pressure. Produce with purple hues contain a variety of polyphenols to support healthy inflammation responses. These veggies also support the urinary tract and liver function. Choose red beets, purple cabbage, red onions, eggplant, purple beans, purple carrots, purple sweet potatoes and purple cauliflower.

Whole fresh fruit (also a carb) can be a star with flavor, sweetness and nutrition for your diet. Fresh fruit is loaded with vitamins, minerals and fiber, especially vitamin C and other antioxidants, potassium, and so much more. Eating a variety of fruit adds diversity of nutrients to your diet.

Ideally fruit should be eaten alone because it digests quickly, using different digestive enzymes. Eating fruit alone lets your body process and assimilate the nutrients efficiently. Fruit combined with other foods won't digest quickly and may begin to ferment in the stomach causing digestive distress. A health supportive goal for eating fruit is one hour before a meal or two hours after a meal. If a meal is particularly heavy, you may have more digestive ease by eating the fruit farther out than two hours after the meal.

If your digestion isn't upset by combining fruit with other foods, indulging in a small bowl of berries or peaches with fresh whipped (dairy or coconut) cream is a yummy treat. Take five minutes to whip real cream (or coconut cream) with a little honey or maple syrup and enjoy this simple but seemingly decadent dessert.

Fresh berries are bursting with the finest nutrition. Stocking up on whole fresh organic berries when in season and freezing in small packages is a great way to be food ready. The frozen fruit can be added to yogurt and smoothies easily. Using non- dairy yogurt, nut milk or coconut milk for fruit smoothies supports similar digestive patterns. Dairy tends to require more digestive effort.

Eat fruit sparingly (just a piece of whole fruit a day or less is ideal) if you have blood sugar regulation issues. Since the glycemic factor or index is a measure of how the food affects blood glucose levels, low glycemic fruits will have a lesser impact on blood glucose. Low glycemic fruits include avocados, apples, cranberries, grapefruit, lemons, limes, pears and plums. Eat the edible fruit skin because it is loaded with nutrition and fiber which will slow the impact of glucose resulting from the fruit. With strong digestion, but wobbly blood sugar, adding some protein like nut butter, nuts or cheese slices to a sliced apple, pear or other low glycemic fruit can be beneficial for steady blood sugar.

Enjoy fruit early in the day. You won't enjoy fruit's natural sugar keeping you awake when you've eaten fruit late in the day or evening. Enjoy pure 100% juice sparingly. Juice causes the blood glucose factor to rise, and sugar is often added to fruit juice drinks.

Considering the naturally high sugar content of dried fruit, enjoy it in small amounts.

Health benefits and nutrition of fruit are akin to the veggies of the same color (described above with veggies). Choose fruit grown closest to home (for ripeness and best nutritional benefits) with a firm feel and a natural essence of its scent to indicate freshness. Bananas, oranges, grapefruit, lemons, limes, avocados, apples of all cultivars and colors, peaches, apricots, grapes, melons, berries, cherries, pineapple, papaya, mango, nectarines, star fruit, kiwi, persimmons, figs, dates, pears, plums and tangerines are among some of the more commonly found fruit in the grocery store.

Note: I didn't intentionally leave out any veggies or fruit. I apologize to those that didn't make the list. You are all good in your own right!

Phytonutrients, also known as phytochemicals, are said to have protective benefits against dis-ease because they are anti-inflammatory and support healthy microbiome, or the good gut bacteria essential to immunity. Phytonutrients include flavanoids, resveratrol, carotenoids and phytoestrogens. Veggies and fruits are rich in phytonutrients.

Fiber is indigestible carbohydrates. The body must eliminate it. Substances not beneficial to the body bind to fiber and are also eliminated. Healthy fiber intake bulks stool which promotes the elimination of waste and prevents constipation.

Harvard's T.H. Chan, School of Public Health describes the two types of fiber:

❖ Soluble fiber, which dissolves in water, can help lower glucose levels as well as help lower blood cholesterol. Foods with soluble fiber include oatmeal, nuts, beans, lentils, apples and blueberries.

❖ Insoluble fiber, which does not dissolve in water, can help food move through your digestive system, promoting regularity and helping prevent constipation. Foods with insoluble fibers include wheat, whole wheat bread, whole grain couscous, brown rice, legumes, carrots, cucumbers and tomatoes.

The best sources of fiber are whole grain foods, fresh fruits and vegetables, legumes, nuts and tea. Adequate fiber (20 – 30 grams per day) also lessens risk for heart disease, type 2 diabetes, breast cancer, diverticular disease and constipation. (https://www.hsph.harvard.edu/nutritionsource/carbohydrates/fiber/) Choose a variety of real food to assure adequate fiber for optimal elimination and wellness.

Microbiome (good gut bacteria) feeds on fiber. The range of healthy balance of microbiome to human cells varies from 1:1 to 10:1. The majority of immunity lives in our gut. When we have adequate fiber intake we are supporting healthy elimination, healthy microbiome and healthy immunity. High fiber diets may reduce the risk of stroke, high cholesterol and potentially heart disease along with supporting healthy blood sugar levels. (http://www.nutritionfacts.org/fiber)

Prebiotics are indigestible fiber that feed probiotics and microbiome. Eating a variety of food should also include prebiotic foods like asparagus, Jerusalem artichokes, legumes, raw chicory root, raw dandelion greens, raw and cooked onions, raw wheat bran and raw banana.

Probiotics are friendly gut bacteria. They support good microbiome balance and are naturally occurring in traditional foods, or result from time honored preparation like soaking, culturing and fermenting. Modern methods of food preservation including cooking at high heat, heavily processing and refining foods, and even soaking poultry in chlorine prior to distribution has put a kibosh on the presence of probiotics in much of our food.

Include probiotic rich foods like raw sauerkraut, kimchi, yogurt without sugar, brine cured olives, raw cheese, kefir, miso, tempeh, kvass and kombucha to support gut health. Begin adding probiotic rich (fermented) foods slowly. Start with just a spoonful, gradually increasing your serving size to two to four ounces one or more times a day. Children may be more willing to try the 'fizzy foods' as opposed to the 'real name'. With children, begin with a single strand or small bite and expose them to more gradually. The palate and digestion will adjust a nice and easy approach.

Probiotic supplementation is also common. When choosing a probiotic supplement, start with a quality brand offering a variety of strains of the cultures. A strain is the bacterium colony or species of the friendly bacteria. Lactobacillus is one of the more common strains. You'll recognize the strains listed on the label by the similarly long names. Choosing a probiotic product with at least five different strains is a good start. People experience varying probiotic results when taken with or without food. Some people have best results taking a probiotic supplement before bed, others prefer probiotics before meals. Experiment and see how you feel with different probiotics at different times of the day if you feel supplementation may be a healthful course for you.

Qualified practitioners may be able to make recommendations based on your symptoms and test you for efficacy of various strains or blends/products. Some people find supplementation effective when immunity is stressed or they are traveling. Probiotics aren't recommended for people with histamine reactions or very sensitive intestinal conditions. Consult with your Physician or qualified practitioner.

Protein & Fat: In the human body and nature (foods people eat), protein and fat are found together. Quality protein and healthy fat work in tandem to generate energy, strength, rejuvenation and other proper function. When someone does not eat animal protein they are wise to consume a wide variety of healthy fats with their sources of protein.

To think a low-fat craze was a common practice intended for health just a couple of decades ago seems ridiculous. As the fat found naturally in foods was replaced with sugar or other unwanted substances to make up for lost taste and structure, the protein was also lost. People are beginning to recognize the harm of a low-fat diet.

Fat is the basis for every healthy human cell. Lipid – that is, fatty - molecules constitute about 50% of the mass of most animal cell membranes, nearly all the remainder being protein. (https:-//www.ncbi.nlm.nih.gov/books/NBK26871/) The importance of ingesting and assimilating quality protein and healthy fat for a healthy human body is of the utmost necessity to assure great function.

Dr. Hyman (2016) says a processed high sugar diet is driving disease and obesity, not fat. His book *Eat Fat, Get Thin: Why the Fat We Eat Is the Key to Sustained Weight Loss and Vibrant Health* details how the myth that fat (and cholesterol) as being detrimental to health has been proliferated under the guise of science and studies. Dr. Hyman (2016) brilliantly describes the studies of old and new as well as putting explicit scientific details about dietary fats in layman's terms. His book is a very detailed guide for including fat as food in a balanced healthful diet.

In order to assimilate the nutritional benefits quality protein and healthy fat offer, digestion must be working well. The best food, undigested, will be of no benefit to the body. Undigested foods can do more harm than good. Refer to Chapter 7 for tips to optimize digestion.

Some of the primary functions of quality protein and healthy fat:
Would you want to give up any of these?

❖ The body needs protein as a building block to assemble proteins needed to form tissue, organs and muscles.

❖ Proteins are catalysts for all biological processes.

❖ Vital to hormonal function and making neurotransmitters.

❖ Chemical messengers for your cells.

❖ Proteins help fight infection

❖ Form red blood cells to oxygenate our blood and virtually every bodily function including metabolism.

❖ Healthy fats are required to absorb vitamins A, D, E and K.

❖ Fats assist energy regulation.

❖ Integral to each and every cell in the body.

❖ Fats protect the organs.

❖ Fats are needed for healthy inflammation and anti-inflammation.

The body needs both inflammation and anti-inflammation processes for optimal wellness and healing. As an example, healthy inflammation occurs when you have an injury and white blood cells rush to the area to protect the injury. Regularly consuming a variety of healthy fats in balance with your body's natural anti-inflammation and inflammation cycles work in tandem to promote healing and homeostasis. Fats out of balance contribute to slow healing. Unhealthy inflammation, out of balance with anti-inflammation, can be the pre-cursor to disease.

Omega 3s (Polyunsaturated Fats "PUFA") - Omega 3 fats tend to be missing from the American diet. Choose more Omega 3 rich oils and foods to balance your Omega 3 to Omega 6 ratio. Ideally the Omega 6:Omega 3 ratio would be about 1:1 in the human body. To know your Omega 3 to Omega 6 ratio get tested by a qualified practitioner or Physician.

Omega 3 fats are good for cardiovascular health and are said to reduce cancer risk. Fish oil, cod liver oil, flaxseed oil, walnut oil and hemp oil are rich sources of Omega 3s. More food sources of Omega 3s include salmon, other fatty fish like tuna, sardines and mackerel, walnuts, chia seeds, sprouted radish seeds, fresh basil and dried oregano. Omegas 3s include EPA and DHA which are good for brain and eye development and health. There may be a link to Alzheimer's prevention with EPA and DHA. If you are prescribed blood thinners consult with your Physician before supplementing Omega 3s.

Omegas 6s (Polyunsaturated Fats 'PUFA') - While it is essential to consume Omega 6 fats because they cannot be made in the body, their consumption in SAD is often out of balance with Omega 3s. Omega 6 fat consumption is compromised by poorly grown (chemicals and modified treated seeds), overly refined oils and rancid products plentiful on store shelves.

Omega 6 fats are found naturally in blackcurrant seed, evening primrose, sunflower oil, pumpkin, and sesame oil (very delicate so choose untoasted). Eggs, poultry, nuts and avocado are good food sources of Omega 6 fats. Check dates on oils and discard faithfully when past date. Omega 6 fats quickly become rancid with heat, moisture, oxygen and require refrigeration for optimal freshness and longevity. To avoid spoiled Omega 6 fats, focus on choosing sources naturally found in real lively food.

Omega 9s (Monounsaturated Fatty Acids 'MUFA') - are unsaturated fats commonly found in vegetable and animal fats. They are relatively stable and thus can be used for gentle heat cooking. They are liquid at room temperature and partly solid when refrigerated. They are especially supportive of cardiovascular health.

Omegas 9 fats are found in extra virgin olive oil, olives, hazelnuts, avocados, nuts, seeds and peanut butter. Considering what appears to be so much mischief and confusion about olive oil sources and inaccurate labeling, be mindful to choose a reliable source. Rely on the USDA organic certification as a good standard for olive oil and choose a dated product in a dark glass bottle for preservation of the oil to a high standard.

Contrary to what is becoming outdated public opinion, saturated fats are vital for health. Cholesterol is a necessary healing agent for arteries and veins. Dietary cholesterol has little to do with the body's cholesterol levels. Saturated fat in moderation is healthful for the liver, vascular system, immunity, aids in calcium absorption and supports healthy cellular structure. Saturated fats are stable at high temperatures. Use them for high heat cooking. Examples include red palm oil, coconut oil, ghee, butter (although butter and ghee will easily burn), and animal fats from pastured animals (like lard or tallow). Duck fat has also come into favored style among foodies and chefs.

Do not eat hydrogenated or partially hydrogenated oils or refined and vegetable oils. They are toxic and interfere with essential roles of healthy fats in the body. Much of the problem with vegetable oils is the extreme processing and refinement they sustain. It isn't uncommon for damaged products to be rancid. Getting rid of oils older than six months is a safe practice to assure integrity of quality. Avoid products with labels that say Refined or Cold Processed which are marketing gimmicks. Choose oils with labels that state Cold Pressed, Expeller Pressed, Unrefined, Unfiltered, Extra Virgin and Organic.

Quality Protein Sources

Fish: Fish can be a lovely complement to a nutritious diet as a delicious protein source. Those who do not eat meat of mammals may find fish palatable. Pregnant women should consult with their Physician before consuming fish.

The question of whether to eat farmed or wild fish is controversial. It is logical to eat wild fish because they live as nature intended, although the ocean is becoming more polluted all the time. One expert I heard from said she will only eat fish from a particular hemisphere. For some, this is too limiting. For others this resonates as a necessary choice. Choosing smaller fish may limit exposure to heavy metals said to accumulate in the tissue of large fish such as tuna, halibut, swordfish and mahi mahi.

Common complaints about farmed fish include: the fish are fed genetically modified ingredients they aren't designed to eat (i.e. corn and soy). According to Pollan (2008) 'we are what we eat eats' so it makes sense to consider the diet of fish same as we consider what is applied to produce or fed to animals raised for consumption. Because farmed fish live in a confined area which may be contaminated with feces, they may require antibiotics. Prey fish, sometimes the diet for farmed fish, may become extinct if they are fed to other fish in excess. Fish farming practices may be considered inhumane. Fish farming may contribute to disease in the wild fish population and damage the environment in other ways. It has also been stated that farmed salmon has lower Omega 3 fats. The pink color is added via dye to farmed salmon rather than the naturally wild pink salmon color.

Grass Fed Beef: According to Mayo Clinic, 'grass fed beef which are given a diet of grass and other foraged foods through their lifetime, may have benefits other types of beef don't have including less total fat; more heart healthy Omega 3 fatty acids; and more conjugated linoleic acid (CLA), a type of fat that's thought to reduce heart disease and cancer risks and more antioxidant vitamins, such as vitamin E.' (http://www.mayoclinic.org/diseases-conditions/heart-disease/expert-answers/grass-fed-beef/FAQ-20058059). Beef raised by conventional (not grass fed) methods generally eat corn. The animal isn't designed by nature to digest grains (and corn) which along with other confined raising techniques, may promote the need for antibiotics and dis-ease to the animal.

More quality protein sources for vital energy creation:

❖ Pastured organic poultry fed a non-vegetarian diet (or at least not 100% vegetarian because poultry naturally eats some protein like bugs).

❖ Pastured lamb raised in a natural setting.

❖ Pastured organic eggs.

❖ Nuts, seeds, beans and legumes that your body digests well.

❖ Protein powders.

Note on protein powders: Many protein powders are combined with artificial ingredients, sugar, preservatives and synthetic nutrients. Pea protein and whey are a couple of the more popular and often 'cleaner' (depending on the maker) varieties. Keep in mind that the protein source is highly refined to become a powder. Some people swear by protein powder and others don't get a great result. Buy small sample packages to allow for cost effective sampling prior to purchasing an entire tub of the product.

Include quality protein with every meal for a basic premise to set you up for having great energy. A quality source of protein about the size of the palm of your hand along with healthy fat is a good starting point. If you are into specific measurements, a protein target for adult women is about 45 – 50 grams (g) per day (more if you are pregnant or breast feeding).

Everyone including women, babies, children, teens and men will vary in amount of optimal daily protein. Activity level also determines protein needs. The elderly must still eat protein several times a day even though their activity is less. Some people experience the source of protein skews the amount needed daily. Although 15 g of a protein is a hefty amount, when delivered via a protein bar, the overall satiation and long burning energy factor may be different than 15 g of a meat source.

Each person will have a unique experience with their protein requirements depending on the kind of protein, their activity levels and overall metabolic needs. As always, use your feelings (energy, satiation, etc.) as a guide for what is right for you. Too much of a good thing can be as disadvantageous as not enough. Find your personalized healthy balance.

H2O

Most of us have plenty of access to pure water, yet many Americans are chronically dehydrated. Americans are dehydrated to epidemic proportions because we drink so much coffee, tea, soda, alcohol, energy and juice drinks instead of water. Consuming healthy beverages other than water in moderation and compensating with more water to balance their dehydrating effects is sensible.

Water is vital for health. The body has many uses for water including regulating body temperature, oxygenation of blood, transporting nutrients, eliminating toxins, and providing electrical communication signals. When you don't drink enough purified water, your body has to prioritize function and something must go undone. Signs of dehydration include thirst, dry mouth, less frequent urination, fatigue, headaches/migraines, muscle cramps, irritability, heartburn, joint pain, confusion and constipation. If you experience any of these discomforts, try drinking adequate water every day for three weeks and see how much better your body feels.

How much H20 is enough? Adequate water consumption is about ½ of the person's body weight in ounces times (X) the ounces of diuretics by 1.5 (not to exceed a gallon of water daily unless advised by a Physician). Alcohol, coffee, soda, fruit juice, energy drinks and some teas are examples of diuretics.

Here is a consumption formula example: If a person weighs 150 lbs and drinks 20 ounces of diuretics = 105 (75 + 30) ounces of purified water daily. Distilled water isn't usually advised, unless Physician recommended.

Beginning the day with a glass of room temperature water is a great way to love your body and mind. Through the night the body and brain have been performing trillions of biochemical and metabolic functions without any hydration. A glass of water upon rising will get your internal terrain moving and restore it in the direction of hydration. Then sipping room temperature water throughout the day, with more before and after exercise is beneficial.

Keep water consumption at meal time to around four ounces to promote digestion. Too much water with meals depletes needed hydrochloric acid and other digestive enzymes. Hold back more water consumption until an hour or so after the meal has passed.

Much of urban water is chlorinated. While chlorination is intended to serve a purpose of keeping water safe until it gets to your home, ingesting chlorine is disruptive to health. Get your water quality tested and you will have the information you need to make a good decision regarding filtration. Filtering water to remove at least chlorine is supportive of wellness. Reverse osmosis filtration removes minerals. If you choose reverse osmosis to filter water, re-mineralization of the water or other mineral supplementation is advised. Get input from a qualified practitioner so your re-mineralization is effective and balanced.

Variety is the Spice of Life

While there can be comfort in the known, variety is indeed the spice of life. Variety implies a wide array of nutrients. Eating a wide selection of food creates more opportunity for the body to get all of the nutrients it needs.

Most people eat a small number (around 10 – 15) of the same foods on an on-going basis. This is boring and limits the nutrition received. Diversifying food choices can range from trying new fresh seasonal produce bursting with ripeness to choosing different varieties of your favorite foods.

Choosing different cultivars of produce gives the benefit of different minerals and nutrients from the soil the crop was grown in. Go ahead and choose different carrots, potatoes, lettuce and other choices typical for you. Then broaden your senses for food and be open to trying new foods.

Create more interest on your plate with an assortment of color. Experiencing more food with your senses gives you delicious variety of texture, taste, smells and sight. Slowing to enjoy the variety and experience of beautiful food in front of you supports optimal digestion, assimilation and absorption of nutrients.

Some nutrients, vital for life, are essential to get from food because the body will not make them. Variety in your diet supports you to receive essentials for the creation of strength and energy from proteins. Ten amino acids (the building blocks of proteins) are considered essential because the body cannot produce them. You must get these from foods or supplementation. Always choose food first. Seek the input of a qualified practitioner (whose business isn't primarily selling amino acid supplements) before supplementing amino acids. Be sure your choice is of pure quality and a good source, and will be effective for your body.

Eat Seasonally

For eons of time, Mother Nature has cued the beasts, critters and even humans to eat in cycles reflecting availability of food (growing seasons) and the creature's energy needs. This masterful design inspires squirrels to stash nuts for winter and bears to come out of hibernation foraging for new crop growth in springtime.

Humans have hunted, gathered, and stored food in preparation for winter; and come out of doors in spring to partake in the freshness of new crops. Since we aren't following hunter and gatherer cycles any longer, mankind doesn't have the need to be nearly as in tune with nature's sync of food crops as it once did. Your body has not changed all that much since the days of ancestral mankind. Choose food in sync with nature's food crop cycles. You will be making choices which resonate with your body's design and natural tendencies.

Springtime is when humans tend to want to shed what they may have gained in the winter. This natural cycle promotes lighter food fare as reflected by seasonally fresh food. In summer humans naturally expend the highest levels of energy, requiring more carbohydrates. Higher glucose production results from higher carbohydrate intake as a quick source of energy for muscles to work. It is no coincidence that summer time harvests produce fruits and vegetables which should serve as your primary carbohydrates. In fall and winter, more of the starchy root crops become available to amplify glucose for energy storage. Traditionally wheat was a fall crop, aiding more energy storage. Higher protein consumption is natural during fall and winter when warming and hearty stews, soups, beef roasts and whole roasted turkeys are desired.

Douillard (2000) eloquently offers his '3-Season Diet' with detailed meal plans and grocery shopping lists to make the process of eating seasonally simple. This diet varies the inclusion of food with nature's seasons. The wide variety of choices suggested in Douillard's '3-Season Diet' lend well to personalizing food choices based on preference and traditional seasonal availability.

Douillard's approach incorporates making choices based on your body type. It may serve as a guide to help you personalize your food life. Doing so, you will honor your body's needs and preferences in sync with your bio-chemistry. Most people aren't strictly one body type. Be aware of your own inclinations and choose foods ideal for your unique self.

While many people may not choose a strict seasonal diet, it is a worthwhile guide to eating for life. The idea of general seasonal eating can evolve in your life and build on a real lively food plan. Lean toward the items you know are traditionally seasonal. Intention to choose food grown closest to home can lend to a natural evolution of eating seasonally. This is a sound practice for wellness.

Chapter 12

Personalize Your Food Life

'To Thine Own Self Be True'

~Shakespeare's Hamlet

Embracing the blessing of being able to choose food you love, you will support your well-being in a basic and fundamental way. Experiencing food as a joy of life to be savored is simply satisfying. Enjoy fueling yourself with delicious real food that makes you feel happy and energized. You deserve to feel good.

For the moment, think of your body as separate from yourself. You've got You; and You need your body for the journey of life. The idea is to think of your body as a means of travel for life. Connect yourself to what your body needs, and You will win as a cohesive YOU (body, mind and spirit). Nourishing your body is a means to get what you want from life. Getting what you want from life starts with feeling your best.

Feeling your best begins with listening to what your body has to say. Feelings are your innate guidance system. Your body communicates its delight, displeasure and even burden with the way you feel.

❖ Feelings are personal clues which tell you where your body is asking for support.

❖ Attending to your feelings is the key to intercept adversity.

❖ Feelings empower every level of wellness.

❖ Feelings will tell you what is right for your body.

It's too common not to be sure of your own feelings. Don't let life; laziness or excuses numb you out. Being mindful of how you feel is the pathway nature laid out for you to know if you are on track with everything in your life. Pain and discomfort are the body's way of saying something isn't right. Honing your skills to listen to your body is a practice worth evolving.

Tapping in to nature's design to eat what your body needs, you can forget the outdated caloric model. This inept model has proven to be an inefficient accounting for how bodies thrive. The human body needs targeted nutrition beyond a caloric unit to match energy. Calories alone don't equate to nourishment.

Cravings are the body's way of asking for something it needs. Douillard (2000) has determined that if your body craves something, it actually needs what it craves – even if that something is inappropriate and ultimately unhealthful! The problem, according to Douillard (2000), is not the craving but the imbalance that has led to the craving.

Getting good exercise is a key to care for you. Everyone should be getting daily adequate movement for cardiovascular health, strength and flexibility training. Find what works for you and do it regularly. Modern lives come with many conveniences which make structured exercise for health of your body and mind a necessity.

Excusing poor food choices because you worked out is a clumsy strategy for weight control or wellness. You can't out exercise poor food choices lacking in nutrition and excelling at adulterated ingredients. Stop 'treating' yourself to junkie food and drink after you have exercised thinking it will be okay because you exercised. Hitting the gym to work off a toxin laden meal is an unskilled approach to self-care. The idea of 'treating' you to anything comprised of junkie ingredients (food or beverage) post workout is nonsensical.

Let Satiation be your Guide

Satiation is a big clue to how well your meals are serving your body. When your meal is nourishing, the body sends signals of satiation. When you begin to feel full, your consumption slows naturally. This way of eating is a result of well-balanced nutrition.

If you feel like you can eat with abandon until your plate or the package is empty, and when you consider what you ate you don't have much to say, begin a practice of simply noticing how your food makes you feel. Life is at its best when you get this skill down.

When you eat a junkie food meal or snack converting to high blood glucose quickly, you want to continue until the food is gone. Each bite tastes as good as the next one. Imagine a package of cookies or crackers where the last one in the bag tastes as good as the first one. Your body isn't becoming satiated because the food is void of nutrition. You are motivated by the chemicals created to taste so good without one iota of nutrition.

Empty calories and high blood glucose set the stage for wanting to eat again soon. Perhaps within a couple of hours or less you will feel 'hunger'. Your body is responding to a need to boost its blood sugar. Frequent eating and grazing stimulates the pancreas to release insulin. Excess glucose is stored as fat and triglycerides. Over time the pancreas can become worn out and unable to release insulin. This is the onset of Type 2 Diabetes. Intervene the onset of dis-ease with your food and drink choices. Mind the stress your body is conveying with signs and symptoms your body expresses.

Hunger without a blood sugar dive feels completely different than the urgent and sometimes scary feeling you get (shaky, headaches, exhaustion and even panic) when you have to eat *right now* to recover your blood sugar. Healthy hunger becomes a thought without urgent alarm that the time to eat is approaching. Find yourself comfortably going four, five and even six hours without eating, and you know your blood sugar patterns are stabilizing. Real lively food is tremendously supportive for healthy blood sugar regulation.

No More Dieting

Imagine a 'cave couple' of ancestral times sitting about making their New Year resolutions to drop the pounds they gained all year (and the year before that and the year before that). Maybe they would make a plan to throw boulders or do laps around the cave, (weather permitting) or jog in place inside the cave. The possibilities for a chuckle on this idea are fun. But I doubt you have you ever seen an image of an obese 'cave couple' or their obese children staring at the cave drawings.

Obesity and dieting culture in America is a modern invention, a result of a damaged food supply and lackadaisical personal choices. It is rather SAD (pun intended) how humans will let themselves go to seed as so many do. This behavior is a reflection of the addictive nature of the food and lifestyle (devices everywhere imposing themselves as entertainment without exercise, as an example).

Diets seem to be attractive and even sexy while you contemplate (and count on) the diet to enter a new realm of being as if a whole new you, free of the burden (usually pounds), will emerge. People prepare for diets, indulging naughtily and freely because they have determined the date their next diet will begin. They proclaim they will tow the mark soon, once their diet begins. They repeat this wishful thinking while they go ahead and consume more of what they know makes them feel and look bad.

Until the diet begins, you will squeeze yourself into your clothes or shift the size up; your eyes aren't clear; you aren't sleeping well; and you eat blindly. Why do people persist in this guilt ridden self-deprecating behavior? Not because they don't 'know better', but because those foods are addicting. Even modern refined gluten making someone sick is addicting.

When you begin a diet, you are ready to relieve your body of the burden you've been taxing it with. Your body may react favorably and you feel lighter. The scale may reflect positivity. Your skin may clear. You may begin to sleep better.

Most diets don't guide people to eat well for the long term. Most diets are a 'one size fits all' approach. One diet isn't right for everyone. Consuming one food deemed healthy, but isn't agreeable for your unique body is detrimental. I've seen it happen with very common foods regarded as healthy like tomatoes and avocados. People can be so consumed by following a regimen of a diet, a well-intentioned plan, that they may miss the cues of the foods not agreeable for them.

Long term premises of low-carb diets and other regimens that limit a large category of food like grains can be harmful when nutrients in quality sources of those foods are eliminated for long periods of time.

Living sustainably in the sense of a personalized food life means choosing food that feels like you are getting what you need from your food. A sustainable food plan is one you truly enjoy without depriving restrictions. A sustainable plan is a way of eating you can live by for weeks, months and years.

By nature, dieting implies deprivation. The rules and restrictions of dieting are not sustainable for a long period of time. You might reach your weight goal. But you can't sustain yourself with the rules and restrictions of dieting. You begin to feel bad because your body isn't getting what it needs. Ultimately, you will break down and succumb to old bad habits and unhealthy cravings that ultimately set you back unless you find your personalized food life. A personalized food life is abundant with choices that are healthy for you.

Not only is it possible to experience being diet-free for a lifetime, but it is a natural result of eating real lively food you love and find delicious and satiating.

Imagine indulging in ice cream, cheesecake, birthday cake, pizza, spaghetti and meatballs…. whatever you like, provided it is made with real food ingredients and consumed in moderation. Your body has the opportunity to naturally heal and age so much more gracefully and beautifully when you aren't dumping toxic ingredients into your precious system.

The nature of life is to ebb and flow. You will certainly get curve balls. Your best laid plans will throw you a zinger. Your best laid plans for your meals will be sidetracked by work deadlines, family emergencies, and bad weather impeding your schedule or availability to get your hands on the food to fulfill your plans. Life happens. Sometimes you simply need a 'super easy do nothing in the kitchen because you don't feel like it break'. Celebrate because it is time for a cheat.

Your body and mind are programmed to thrive with real lively food input. Find pleasure in real food. Whether you are putting grass fed butter on a beautiful piece of warm sourdough bread, eating a homemade cookie of the finest ingredients, sharing a decadent dessert with a friend, or something else you find a treat, ENJOY every bite. Savor the texture and taste and aroma. Feel the enjoyment of beautiful real food.

The combination of moderation, real lively ingredients and pleasure will keep you on your wellness path.

Be Cheat Ready

Having a cheat list ready will soften the inevitable idea that every day won't be perfect. The idea is to be prepared so cheating doesn't leave you falling hard or slipping into an old bad rut.

Remember, ingredients matter. If you reach for an old bad habit look at what's in it. Be grounded in a commitment to allow yourself real food at all times. There is always a better option than junkie food. If you are inclined to fall for a bad choice, choose a better option. For example: If cookies are your weakness and life circumstances have brought you to the cookie aisle of your 'super' market, resist the old bad habit. Scoot on over to a cookie with more favorable ingredients.

Read the label and confirm the ingredients are agreeable for you. You may find a good replacement for a 'bad cookie' replacement in the refrigerated snack section where fresher (preservative free) items are located. This is where more 'artisanal' brands are often located. Maybe a coconut based truffle will satisfy your body, mind and spirit.

If the vending machine is really your only choice, then get that 'cookie'. Savor it and eat that 'cookie' slowly. Give yourself messages to be in the present moment, mindfully aware of how that 'cookie' makes you feel. You may feel relief if your hunger was pervasive. Above all don't be hard on yourself for eating a 'bad cookie'. Move on.

Choose the best cheat you can afford Make a cheat an opportunity to treat yourself to something you love, whether it is a special restaurant with a fantastic menu based on real foods prepared in house, or a delicious real food ingredient pizza, or something else, mark the day as the break you need to recharge. Use the cheat as a reprieve, as an investment to feed your soul in a way vacation refreshes you.

Never make a choice that will harm your body. Celiac diagnosed people should not eat gluten as a treat, for example. Food sensitivities and allergies must always be honored. Let common sense prevail.

Rejoice in your transformation! You will know you are making the greatest strides for your health when you take a bite or sip of something formerly very familiar (that old bad habit) in your regular diet (soda, snack foods, fast food, etc) and it makes you a feel a little nauseas. It will be so distasteful you will get rid of it and wonder how you ever managed to function eating that junk. The body amazingly compensates for your bad choices. In reality, it was fighting back and sacrificing proper function to keep you going. Now that you've peeled back the distress to find your true vibrant self, your body will resist negative input.

Personalizing your food life is a means to find a wellness groove that fits your body, mind and life. Eating healthfully and loving your food while living a busy modern life full of its fantastic inventions and conveniences can still be yours. Just don't choose invented food. When food is too convenient (the old saying too good to be true) it really isn't a good thing. Choose wisely for you; choice by choice day after day.

Be Mindful. Create conscious attention about what you are going to eat and drink. Make food plans and be food ready with the guidance offered in this book. Keep a cheat list nearby. Keep focus and consider your best options to go off 'the rails' a bit without being self-destructive when life calls for you to go off your food plans.

Ideas for your cheat list:

❖ Have a few gluten free, farm to table or other special restaurants offering quality food.
❖ Include a couple of take out options. (Like Chipotle Mexican Grill or Tokyo Joe's in my area).
❖ Include restaurant options close to home, school and work.
❖ Include the best restaurant in your town where you would like to dine, but haven't (yet).
❖ Acceptable cheat food at home (Like a gluten free minimal real food ingredient pizza).

❖ Quick snack foods to relieve temptation for a former vice. Keep them in close reach in your desk, car and pantry. Change up your choices so you don't get bored. Reference the snack list in Chapter 10.

Repel drama. Taking an occasional break from your new normal is your new normal. Be aware of your present moment - mindful of what you are eating and how it makes you feel while you are savoring each bite. This is your cheat so be especially mindful of the moment. Take in the smell, taste, texture and how much you are enjoying a break. Enjoy yourself.

Live in Your New Normal

Keep evolving food choices with real food that tastes fantastic and loves your body. This new normal is personally appealing and sustainable for your life. Become firmly planted in the practice of making healthful choices as the basis for how you live your life.

Easy sustainable steps reinforce new behavior for lasting results. Solidifying new behavior into regular routines takes about 21 days of consistent practice. Be persistent with easy steps to create new habits and routines which give your life wellness. Build layer upon layer of healthy habits as a foundation for a lifestyle which truly nourishes you.

Chapter 13

Yummy Recipes Free of Gluten

"I'm just someone who likes cooking and for whom sharing food is a form of expression."

~Maya Angelou

The 19 recipes I've put together for you are from my personal arsenal of favorite recipes I've created. They are what I consider basic recipes, all easy and with options for you to adjust for your personal preference. I like to think of them as 'All American (Real) Food Fare'. They are all free of gluten and meant to launch and expand your personal wellness journey with food as its foundation. I hope you enjoy them as much as I do!

How do you say Bon Appetit! (In English)…
Good Appetite! Enjoy your Meal!

Smoothie with Cranberry & Coconut Milk

Enjoy this whole food nutrient packed drink as a yummy addition to breakfast or lunch or as a snack.

INGREDIENTS:

¼ cup coconut milk from the can
(get the one without guar gum)

1 cup unsweetened almond or other nut milk

1/8 cup fresh cranberries

1 heaping tablespoon canned pumpkin

½ frozen banana

2 pitted medjool dates

Few baby kale or spinach leaves

Spices to taste: cinnamon, nutmeg or cardamom

DIRECTIONS:

Add all to your blender and give it a good spin. Delicious!

Add a pinch of spices to your taste.

Lemon Rosemary Drop Scones

Perfect when you want to indulge in a baked good, make your own to control the ingredients and avoid chemical additives, preservatives and other unwanted ingredients common in commercial products. Lemon Rosemary Drop Scones are made with protein rich real food, designed to be easier on blood sugar regulation than commercially baked goods made wheat or white flour as the leading ingredient. Lemon Rosemary Drop Scones aren't rolled out, saving you time and cleaning.

INGREDIENTS:

½ cup chopped walnuts

1 cup amaranth or spelt flour (amaranth is the gluten free choice)

½ cup oat flour (certified gluten free)

¼ cup almond flour

2 tsp aluminum free baking powder

½ tsp sea or mineral salt

4 Tbsp cold unsalted butter (ideally grass fed)

¼ cup whole fat cow or goat's milk

1 egg

Zest of 1 lemon, about 2 Tbsp

2 Tbsp fresh rosemary chopped

1/3 cup maple syrup + 2 Tbsp for topping

DIRECTIONS:

Preheat oven to 350 degrees.

Line a baking sheet with parchment.

In a large glass bowl combine the flours with a whisk; Add baking powder and salt; Whisk lightly to combine.

Dice cold butter and add to flour mixture using a pastry cutter; Combine until evenly mixed and butter size is crumbly as close to bread crumbs as possible.

In a separate glass bowl whisk milk, egg, lemon zest, maple syrup and rosemary until well combined.

Fold the liquid mixture into the dry mixture until well combined; until all is wet and evenly distributed; careful not to over mix.

Fold in walnuts.

Using a couple of tablespoons, drop dough on the parchment; when they are about two inches in diameter; you'll get about nine scones on a sheet.

With a pastry brush, give the tops a swipe of maple syrup.

Bake about 12 - 15 minutes until golden on top and easily lifted with a spatula and have a light golden color underneath.

Exact baking time will vary with the size of your scones, altitude and oven so keep an eye on them to be just right, and lightly golden on the bottom.

Place on a wire rack, let cool slightly, serve slightly warm.

Store in the refrigerator; can be frozen for a few weeks, IF you have any left! Reheat in a low oven 150 – 200 degrees for about 5 minutes until warmed.

Pumpkin Pancakes

Pumpkin pancakes are a great choice to make ahead and put extra in the freezer for a quick thaw and fast weekday breakfast. Top with an egg or two; generous smear of nut butter or other quality protein (nitrate free bacon, ham or sausage) and you have a fast satisfying breakfast.

INGREDIENTS:

1 cup ancient grain organic Spelt OR Amaranth flour (Amaranth is the gluten free choice)

1 tsp baking soda

1/8 tsp finely ground sea or mineral salt

2 Tbsp gluten free oat bran (or grind gluten free oats in coffee grinder dedicated to seeds, etc)

1 cup whole organic milk or unsweetened non-dairy milk as needed; whole milk works best

¼ cup pumpkin puree (can also substitute with applesauce, butternut squash or sweet potato puree)

2 tsp walnut oil + more for cooking pan

1 large egg, lightly beaten

Maple syrup or honey gently warmed

Real grass fed butter – a tbsp pat for each serving

DIRECTIONS:

Combine the first four ingredients in a large glass bowl.

Combine milk, pumpkin (or butternut or sweet potato), walnut oil and egg in separate glass bowl; stirring to combine then gently whisking until ingredients are incorporated.

Add the liquid mixture to the dry ingredients; stirring / folding until dry ingredients are just moistened (don't over mix)

If using non-dairy milk and the batter appears too thin, add a tablespoon or two more flour; and gently combine.

Let batter rest five minutes before 'griddling'.

Heat griddle or skillet; add walnut oil and bring to medium heat.

The first pancake is always a 'tester' for me. It doesn't usually flip well, so if this happens to you too, just put a scant one 1/8 cup batter pour in first; the remaining pancakes have a better result.

Sizing your pancakes with a ¼ cup of batter is about right to make them easy to turn and fitting several on the griddle. If you feel adventurous try making other shapes (such as Mickey or Minnie Mouse) by putting batter into a squeeze tube.

Griddle pancakes until edges start to bubble and they gently lift; you'll see the golden brown color underneath.   Serve Warm with toppings!

Quinoa Porridge

Quinoa Porridge is a satisfying replacement for oatmeal or any other hot and cold cereal.

INGREDIENTS:

1 cup organic quinoa rinsed in a fine mesh strainer

2 cups purified water

1 cup chopped raw or properly dehydrated nuts: pecans, almonds & walnuts work well

Whole milk or unsweetened non-dairy milk such as coconut or nut milk

Honey or maple syrup

DIRECTIONS:

Add quinoa to water, bring to boil and turn down to simmer; Cover.

Keep on medium heat for about 20 – 25 minutes until all water is absorbed.

Fluff with fork, place 1/2 cup in serving bowl.

Add desired amount of milk, top with nuts and a drizzle of honey or maple syrup.

Serve with a protein like eggs, nitrate free sausage or ham.

Eggs Florentine

This recipe for Eggs Florentine is easy to double for more diners. The key to light and fluffy eggs and preserving the delicate nutrients is cooking them low and slow. Eggs Florentine is delicious for breakfast, lunch or dinner.

INGREDIENTS:

Four pastured eggs (use soy free if you can get them)

3 Tbsp. sour cream or crème fraiche

Two cups baby spinach

¾ cup shredded cheese – Cheddar & Baby Swiss work nicely

Sea salt

1 Tbsp butter

DIRECTIONS:

Whisk eggs in medium size bowl.

Add sour cream or crème fraiche and whisk until well blended and fluffy.

Add pinch of sea salt.

Heat medium skillet to medium heat; and add butter.

Add eggs to melted butter in skillet; turn heat down to medium low and let eggs begin to set a minute or so; gentle shifting of the pan will reveal they are setting slightly.

Gently stir egg mixture over medium low heat until they are nearly done. Low and slow cooking requires patience; you'll love the light and fluffy reward.

When nearly done fold in spinach and continue stirring gently until the spinach is wilted.

Sprinkle the cheese and give a few folds to incorporate and melt the cheese.

Serve piping warm with allowable grain buttered toast if desired. Add a dollop of just fruit jam or honey if desired.

This is delicious with *Nourishing Traditions* Turkey Breakfast Sausage recipe.

Grilled Lemon Chicken

This summertime classic and couldn't be easier for dinner. Lemon Grilled Chicken makes excellent leftovers, sliced over a bed of salad greens and vegetables or as a chicken salad cut in cubes with clean mayo, celery, grapes, and walnuts. As a main dish it pairs nicely with grilled veggies.

INGREDIENTS:

6 Tbsp fresh lemon juice

4 Tbsp extra virgin olive oil

2 garlic cloves, minced finely or tsp garlic granules

Skinless boneless chicken breast halves (this recipe covers about four); If cooking more, adjust the marinade

1/2 tsp sea or mineral salt

1/2 tsp freshly ground black pepper if desired

Scallions to dress the top if desired

DIRECTIONS:

Whisk the first three ingredients in a small glass bowl.

Put the chicken two at a time into a large zip plastic bag; don't seal the bag, but hold it somewhat upright; this allows air to move so you don't pop the bag and keeps juices inside.

Gently pound chicken in the bag with smooth side of a kitchen mallet until even thickness, a few minutes; remove and repeat until done.

Add the marinade to the large zip-top plastic bag with all of the chicken (about 4 to a bag).

Seal the bag. Move it around a bit to cover the chicken with all combined ingredients. Marinate in refrigerator at least 30 minutes (all day is fine too!); turn the bag a few times while marinating.

Brush grill grates and lightly oil them. Heat the grill to medium high.

Place marinated chicken on grill.

Lightly salt & pepper. Baste a little extra marinade on the chicken now, but then discard the marinade bag since it has raw chicken juices (don't marinate at the end of cooking).

Keep an eye on the grill, lowering heat to medium. Don't let it flame up. When you can lift a chicken breast easily with tongs, it is ready to turn.

While still on the grill, place a scallion sliced the long way on the chicken so it sort of fans out.

Grill about 6 minutes on each side or until internal temperature is 165 degrees. After the last flip use a clean utensil to remove so the uncooked chicken juices don't transfer.

Let rest about 5 minutes before cutting. Delish!

Broccoli & Beef Stir Fry

This recipe for Broccoli & Beef Stir Fry is reminiscent of the most flavorful and tender restaurant version, made with the freshest fresh ingredients and grass fed beef; and without any chemicals, excitotoxins (like MSG) or preservatives.

INGREDIENTS:

3 Tbsp gluten free thickener like tapioca starch (arrowroot not advised because it gels)

2 Tbsp plus 1/2 cup purified water

1 - ½ tsp garlic granules (to taste)

1 lb boneless grass fed round steak or New York strip steak cut into thin strips, about 3 inches in length

2 Tbsp coconut oil, divided

4 cups fresh broccoli florets

1 small yellow or white onion cut in wedges

1/3 cup tamari or coconut aminos (the aminos will give a slightly sweeter flavor)

2 Tbsp honey

1- 2 tsp ground ginger (to taste)

2 cups hot cooked rice (1 cup dry rice) and 2 cups water or broth for cooking; (Rice can be soaked in water for 6-8+ hours for sensitive digestion)

DIRECTIONS:

Rinse 1 cup rice and add to pan with 2 cups purified water or broth. Cook according to package directions while preparing beef and broccoli.

In a glass bowl, combine 2 Tbsp gluten free thickener, 2 Tbsp water and garlic granules; blend until smooth.

Add beef and toss to coat with mixture.

Heat large cast iron skillet or wok over medium high heat; add coconut oil.

When oil is melted, add beef evenly around pan.

Lower heat to medium, continue cooking beef low and slow to preserve nutrients.

Turn beef until evenly done.

Remove beef and gently keep warm.

Add broccoli and onion to pan; stir fry for about 5 minutes until done.

Whisk tamari, honey, ginger, 1 Tbsp gluten free thickener and ½ cup water until well combined while broccoli and onion are cooking.

Broccoli should remain bright green and the onion will be slightly soft.

Return beef to pan with broccoli and onion.

Add tamari mixture to pan; stir fry over medium heat for another few minutes until all is piping hot.

Serve over hot rice.

Pork Carnitas

Delicious served over rice, quinoa, in a gluten free wrap or over salad greens. Great as a breakfast leftover dish paired with an egg or two for energy to start a travel day or outdoor adventure or when you just know you need extra fuel for what's ahead.

INGREDIENTS:

1 lb pastured boneless pork chops

1 cup gluten free flour blend

½ tsp thyme, oregano, chili powder, marjoram, salt and pepper; or use a 'clean' (no gluten, no preservatives, additives, sugar etc.) taco seasoning blend

Red pepper, diced (about ½ a cup)

Green onions, bunch, sliced thin to include some greens

½ cup cooked black or adzuki beans

Coconut oil

Fresh mixed greens – about 4 cups

Two avocados diced

Fresh lime sliced or lime juice

DIRECTIONS:

Dice pork into ¼ inch cubes.

Put flour in glass bowl & mix in spices.

Dredge diced pork cubes in flour.

Heat cast iron skillet to medium high; add coconut oil.

Put pork in hot skillet.

Stir with spatula to evenly cook.

When the pork begins to turn golden, add red pepper, green onions and black beans.

Continue cooking, stirring occasionally until pork is all golden and no longer pink in center; and veggies and beans are warm and tender, about 5 more minutes.

Serve over bed of mixed greens and topped with avocado and squeeze of lime.

Crispy Tender Chicken

Here's the answer to your (inner) child's call for 'chicken fingers'. The chicken is tender and juicy. Pair it with any veggie in your crisper drawer; raw, steamed or roasted. Reheated Crispy Tender Chicken is a great breakfast .

INGREDIENTS:

1 lb package boneless skinless chicken thighs cut inch wide strips

1 cup gluten free flour blend

1 cup almond flour

Spices: 1 tsp each: oregano, chili powder, cilantro, fine sea salt, pepper, and paprika

Change/add/delete or omit spices for your diner's preferences

2 eggs

Coconut oil

DIRECTIONS:

Preheat oven to 375 degrees.

In one bowl, combine the gluten free flour blend with 1/2 spice blend.

In second bowl, whisk the eggs.

In third bowl combine almond flour and other 1/2 spice blend.

Heat large cast iron skillet over medium high heat. Add 4 Tbsp coconut oil to melt.

In assembly line fashion, with tongs or fork, take chicken strip and dredge in flour blend, then egg and finish with spiced almond flour.

Put in skillet, keeping space between chicken strips for even cooking. Plan a couple of batches .

Repeat until all are done, turning chicken when golden brown, after a few minutes.

When all chicken pieces are flipped, let them brown to a nice golden color, a few minutes longer.

Place cast iron skillet in pre-heated oven.

Done when reaches internal temperature of 165, about 15 minutes.

Remove with metal spatula to keep the crispy coating will be intact.

Carrots & Peas

Kids are drawn to the natural sweetness of Carrots & Peas. When you want to involve your kids in meal preparation this is an easy choice.

INGREDIENTS:

1 cup fresh or frozen sweet peas (shelled if fresh)

3 large carrots (Mix it up with yellow, orange and purple carrots if available)

2 Tbsp butter

2 Tbsp extra virgin olive oil

DIRECTIONS:

Put peas in small saucepan.

Peel and slice carrots in thin discs.

Add carrots to saucepan.

Add a small amount of water, about ¼ cup.

Bring to simmer over medium heat.

Turn heat to low medium and add butter.

Stir, cover and cook a few minutes.

The carrots should still be firm (overcooking depletes nutrition) and peas cooked through to warm.

Remove from heat when done.

Using a slotted spoon, transfer to plate or serving bowl.

Drizzle extra virgin olive oil & serve.

Kale Salad

Kale salads are great keepers, lasting for days to come. A lettuce or other delicate green salad can't offer comparable lasting freshness. Putting together a Kale Salad with an array of colorful seasonal veggies on a day off work is a healthy addition to your food life.

Properly preparing kale is the key to reap its great nutritive value including vitamins, K, A, E, C, B6, manganese, copper and more plus making it delicious. Choose baby kale for a much milder flavor than a fully mature kale leaf. Clean and spin dry kale leaves. Then chop to desired size and gently massage the kale by itself for a minute or two in a glass bowl. This begins the enzymatic release which mellows the flavor, and begins the slight breakdown of the fibers making it more digestible and therefore increases the nutrient uptake.

Add a simple protein such as baked chicken breast, grilled thinly sliced grass fed beef steak, or grilled/broiled/baked wild fish. Kale salads work well in lunch boxes and even at breakfast with an egg on the side.

One of my favorite Kale Salad combinations is baby kale, thinly sliced French breakfast radish, baby zucchini with grated carrots and a sprinkle of shaved parmesan. This recipe will be your guide while you find your favorite veggie combinations.

INGREDIENTS:

Bunch of kale cleaned with ribs cut off or four or five cups baby kale. Pick the freshest cultivars of kale: Red, Lacitino, Dinosaur, etc.

2 Tbsp lemon juice

3 Tbsp olive oil

Clove of garlic or two, to taste OR ½ - 1 tsp garlic granules

Handful of thinly sliced zucchini – about ½ to 1 cup

Red and yellow bell pepper diced, about ½ to 1 cup

½ cup feta cheese or fresh shaved parmesan

¼ cup toasted pepitos (pumpkin seeds), chopped walnuts or slivered almonds

¼ cup apple sweetened/sugar free dried cranberries or chopped medjool dates

Sea salt

DIRECTIONS:

Rinse and chop the kale into about 1 inch pieces, place in large glass bowl.

Clean and prepare other vegetables; and set aside.

Whisk lemon juice, olive oil, add pinch of sea salt, chopped garlic or garlic granules in small bowl. Set aside for flavors to meld.

In a large glass bowl, gently massage kale with very clean hands until it begins to wilt, a minute or two.

Fold in other vegetables.

Pour dressing over top and stir to evenly coat.

Once served, sprinkle cheese and nuts (fresh option so they don't get soggy, especially if keeping leftovers).

Let the salad come to room temperature if chilled before serving.

Berry Green Summer Salad

Fresh ingredients in Berry Green Summer Salad speak for themselves. This salad is so fresh it almost sparkles!

INGREDIENTS:

1 cup fresh basil leaves – loosely packed and cut thin – chiffonade style/in ribbons

5 cups greens cut or torn in bite sized pieces. Use red or green leaf lettuce, romaine or spinach

Adding a cup of arugula will add a zesty kick. (optional)

2 cups thinly sliced red cabbage

2 cups fresh berries; raspberries, blueberries and blackberries all work very well in this recipe

1 small red onion, sliced thinly

Sea or mineral salt

Goat cheese in small bite chunks

DRESSING INGREDIENTS:

1/3 cup champagne vinegar

1/3 cup sesame (not toasted) oil or extra virgin olive oil

1 Tbsp honey

DIRECTIONS:

Combine all dressing ingredients in glass jar. Shake to combine and let sit while making salad for ingredients to meld; Shake again before serving.

Arrange salad ingredients on a large platter or in a large glass bowl and toss gently. This salad is so pretty, it makes a gorgeous presentation on a platter or clear glass bowl. It is beautiful arranged like a cobb salad, so each diner may take what they desire.

Drizzle the dressing over the salad and season lightly with salt and freshly ground pepper as desired.

Red Cabbage & Carrot Slaw

This vibrant salad, full of flavor and crunch is a good keeper; and packs well in lunch boxes as well as being a delicious addition to a quick workday breakfast.

INGREDIENTS:

½ medium red cabbage head, shredded

5 large carrots, about 1 ½ cups shredded

½ cup raisins, golden or dark; or substitute fruit juice sweetened dried cranberries or cherries

3 Tbsp fresh cilantro or parsley finely chopped

3 Tbsp olive oil

3 Tbsp lemon juice

½ tsp honey

Sea or mineral salt

1/2 tsp dried ginger or ¼ tsp fresh grated ginger

Hemp hearts

DIRECTIONS:

Whisk lemon juice, olive oil, honey and ginger and a dash of sea salt in small glass bowl.

Put vegetables except cilantro or parsley in large glass bowl; and gently stir to combine.

Pour dressing over vegetables; fold in gently to cover all the veggies with dressing.

Add raisins and cilantro or parsley.

Best when chilled before serving so flavors have blended (let come to room temperature a bit before serving).

Sprinkle with hemp hearts just before serving.

Warm Spinach and Beet Salad

This salad is especially delicious in early spring when veggies are bursting out. Serve with crumbled bacon, or top with baked or grilled sliced chicken or a salmon filet.

INGREDIENTS:

6 cups baby spinach

2 Tbsp walnut oil

1 Tbsp maple syrup

1 Tbsp apple cider vinegar

2 tsp grainy brown mustard

2 tsp tamari

Sea or mineral salt

2 cups steamed beet wedges, cut again into one inch cubes (after steamed). Or use packaged pre- cooked beets in shrink wrap (get the one that is just beets/no extra sugar or ingredients)

1 cup of thinly sliced (halved) seeded and peeled cucumber (optional)

¼ cup crumbled goat or feta cheese

1/8 cup chopped walnuts

DIRECTIONS:

To steam beets, remove tops (save for a stir fry or steaming when they are intact), scrub with veggie brush; cut in wedges, put in steamer basket over boiling water, steam about 25 - 30 minutes until just fork tender; do not overcook.

Whisk walnut oil, maple syrup, ACV, mustard, tamari, and pinch of salt in large glass bowl; reserve 2 Tbsp. for the finish.

Add spinach and cucumber to the bowl and toss to coat with dressing. Top with beets, and lightly toss.

Place a serving portion on the plate, top with walnuts and cheese and drizzle with reserved dressing.

Guacamole

Guacamole works as a yummy dip for veggies, brown rice tortilla 'chips', home baked crackers, veggie chips or organic blue corn chips prepared in coconut oil. Guacamole is a good spread on sandwiches and wraps. It's also a great topping for chili, tacos and scrambled eggs. This Guacamole recipe will satisfy you with zippy flavor and freshness!

INGREDIENTS:

3 ripe avocados

3 tsp red chili flakes

2 tsp lemon juice

Sea or Himalayan salt finely ground

DIRECTIONS:

Cut avocado lengthwise and remove pit; scoop the fruit into a medium size glass bowl

Mash with a fork

Add lemon juice and stir. The lemon juice adds brightness and will also help prevent browning of the fruit due to oxidation.

Add red chili flakes, more or less to taste; stir.

Add a pinch or two of the salt to taste.

Bean Dip

Bean Dip is a delicious and nutritious add on to snacks with protein and fiber. Serve with raw veggies; organic corn tortillas, sprouted or rice tortillas with salsa; and beet or sweet potato chips. Bean dip inside a wrap adds extra satisfaction. It is good on toast for breakfast.

INGREDIENTS:

1 can (15 oz.) organic beans rinsed and drained – Black, Adzuki, & Fava Beans all work well. If you've got the time to soak and cook dried beans you will be a leg up nutrition-wise. When using canned beans, opt for a can with a BPA free liner and use the newest stock on the store shelves (and rotate your pantry).

1 – 2 cloves chopped garlic

1 small red onion chopped

2 - 3 tsp olive oil

¼ tsp ground cumin

1/8 tsp cayenne or chili powder blend

Sea salt

3 Tbsp lime juice

¼ cup fresh cilantro chopped

1/8 cup organic tahini (sesame seed paste you will find near nut butters in your grocery store)

DIRECTIONS:

Blend beans, onion, garlic, juice and tahini in food processor until smooth.

Add spices to taste and dash of sea salt and pulse to gently blend.

Slowly add oil through feed tube.

Taste test and adjust with spices or anything else desired.

Put in serving bowl, top with cilantro or parsley if desired.

Tortillas can be heated on baking stone at 350 degrees for about five minutes until crispy and broken into chips for a truly baked chip.

Refrigerates well for a few days.

Pecan Shortbread Cookies

Pecan Shortbread Cookies are a little bite of heaven, melting in your mouth in the most scrumptious way.

INGREDIENTS:

2 cups almond flour

1/8 tsp fine sea salt

6 Tbsp grass fed butter

3 Tbsp maple syrup

¼ tsp vanilla

6 Tbsp chopped raw pecans

DIRECTIONS:

Preheat oven to 350 degrees.

Combine almond flour and salt in small glass bowl.

Combine butter, maple syrup and vanilla in large bowl. Use a mixer for this to get nice and creamy.

Add almond flour and salt mixture to the 'buttery bowl'; stir until you have a cookie dough consistency.

Stir in pecans.

Use teaspoons to form small rounded cookies on parchment line baking sheet.

Dip a fork in a glass of water and give the little cookie a criss-cross pattern.

Bake for about 10 minutes until golden on bottom; watch closely so they don't burn.

Let cool on cookie sheet for 5 – 10 minutes before removing to wire rack.

Store in refrigerator.

Chocolaty Chocolate Chip Cherry Cookies

Antioxidant rich cacao, cherries, almond flour and walnut combination in this recipe offers a gluten free treat and healthy energy boost. This recipe makes about 30 cookies. Store them in a tightly sealed container in the refrigerator to keep them fresh.

INGREDIENTS:

2 ¾ cups blanched almond flour

½ tsp fine sea salt

½ tsp baking soda

½ tsp tapioca starch

¼ cup 100% cacao powder

½ cup walnut oil

½ cup honey

1 Tbsp vanilla extract

¾ cup unsweetened cacao chips. Or use the same amount of coarsely chopped dark chocolate (70% + cacao). I like the chips because I don't have another step of chopping chocolate which is usually messy in my kitchen.

1 cup dried fruit juice sweetened cherries

½ cup chopped walnuts

DIRECTIONS:

Preheat the oven to 350 degrees. Line a baking sheet with parchment paper.

In a large bowl, combine the almond flour, salt, baking soda. Make sure the almond flour doesn't have any clumps. Add cacao powder by pushing it through a stainless steel mesh strainer with a spoon. This prevents lumps and subsequent over mixing. Gently whisk all ingredients until combined.

In another bowl, whisk together the walnut oil, honey and vanilla extract. Use a big measuring cup, topping off with each ingredient as you go. It saves another bowl to wash.

Fold the chocolate, cherries and walnuts into the wet mixture.

Spoon a couple of tablespoons of the dough to form a cookie on the baking sheet. These cookies hold their shape well. A dozen fit nicely on a sheet.

Begin checking for doneness at 8 minutes. They are ready when they lift off the paper easily with a spatula and are very light brown on the bottom. These tend to be somewhat chewy out of the oven.

Banana Cake

This banana cake is a throwback to a frozen 'Sara Lee' cake I loved as a kid. The optional cream cheese frosting recipe that follows makes it extra special. It serves up nicely with a brunch or as an after school/afternoon snack. The moist delicious flavor gives you the delight of sweet satisfaction without jolting blood sugar.

INGREDIENTS:

3 cups almond flour

½ tsp fine sea salt

½ tsp tapioca starch

1 tsp baking soda

¼ cup walnut oil

¼ cup honey

3 eggs

1 Tbsp vanilla

1 large bananas - very ripe (but not brown) – to make about 1/2 cup mashed

¼ cup unsweetened carob chips

¼ cup chopped walnuts (optional)

DIRECTIONS:

Preheat oven to 350 degrees.

Grease a 9-inch round cake pan with a little walnut oil.

In a large glass bowl, combine almond flour, salt, tapioca starch and baking soda. Use a whisk to be sure the almond flour doesn't have clumps.

In a 2-cup glass measuring cup or small bowl, whisk together the walnut oil, honey, eggs and vanilla.

Using the measuring cup lets you add ingredients on top of each other and reduce more bowls to clean.

Fold the wet mixture into the almond flour until thoroughly combined.

Fold in banana and thoroughly combine. Don't over mix, just combine until dry ingredients are moistened.

Fold in carob chips.

Fold in walnuts if using.

Pour into cake pan and smooth out for even distribution.

Bake for 20 minutes; begin checking center for doneness until toothpick inserted in center comes out clean.

Cool in pan on wire rack, cut in wedges to serve. Store in refrigerator.

Cream Cheese Frosting:

Chill a mixing bowl and wire whip attachment in the freezer for 20 minutes.

Let an 8 ounce bar of cream cheese or Neufchatel come to room temperature.

Place the cream cheese in the mixing bowl and bring to high speed, beating the cream cheese until light and fluffy. While the machine is running add a Tbsp or two of maple syrup. Keep whipping until well incorporated.

You are ready to frost your banana cake!

Conclusion

Sow the seeds of uplifting your nutrition by starting where you are now. Small steps practiced consistently create sustained habits and propel great opportunities for wellness.

Listen to what your body is trying to reveal to you.

Rejoice where you are now because you are listening to the call of your body.

Listen to your body's great wisdom because there is only one of you.

Find real lively food to be one of the great joys of life. Choosing food personally appealing for your body, mind and spirit gives you power to fuel your life for wellness.

Listen to how your body and mind feel, to discover which food choices are healthy for you. You set the stage for wellness tomorrow and years down the road.

The interconnected nature of your body resembles that of this amazing planet. Relish the interconnected life shared with one another. Honor the design of life by choosing real food, unadulterated and as close as nature intended. Good choices flow for the benefit of the planet and all of the creatures and plant life inhabiting it.

Be Your Beautiful Self,

Tam John

About the Author

Tam John is a certified Holistic Nutritionist (NTP) with a passion for guiding people to know which choices are healthy for them. She imparts, you can't make healthful choices until you know which choices are healthy for you.

For nearly 30 years, Tam John has been a business development leader and entrepreneur. She founded and was President of an elite Technical Consulting and Executive Recruitment firm as the capstone in her corporate career. From her own personal health crisis and journey back to wellness, Tam found the restorative power of real food right for her body. Tam learned not all 'healthy' food is healthy for everyone. She learned the human body is a seemingly miraculous system of communication that relays where it is stressed and burdened. Tam learned that food and lifestyle directs the course of wellness when genetic tendencies exist. One diet is not right for everyone. Choosing healthy food is a lifestyle practice that can eliminate ever dieting again, while looking and feeling great.

Tam's passion is guiding people to a lifestyle of wellness that works for any contemporary life. Tam's nutritional therapy practice can be found at www.TamJohn.com. She consults with people 1:1 via phone, video and in-person in Colorado. Tam speaks to community and corporate groups about wellness. She expresses how everyone has within them amazing healing and restorative capabilities; and how to find a path to greater wellness whatever the person's health status. She is a regular contributor to *Thrive Global* and writes healthy articles for health/wellness, cooking and financial services companies. *A Fresh Wellness Mindset* is the first book Tam has authored.

Please visit www.TamJohn.com

Resources

https://www.beyondceliac.org/

Awareness, advocacy and action are stated in the logo. Tips to live gluten free

https://celiac.org/

Celiac Disease Foundation site with information about living gluten free, Celiac disease and its signs and symptoms

http://celiac-disease.com/gluten-free-restaurants/

Celiac news and gluten free diet resources

http://celiacrestaurantguide.com/gf-menus/chains-2/

Chain restaurants offering gluten free choices

http://www.doortodoororganics.com

Grocery delivery including perishables for Kansas City, Des Moines, Michigan Chicago, Colorado, New Jersey, Philadelphia. This list may not be inclusive

http://farmshares.info/

Guide to find CSAs in Colorado, Wyoming and Idaho

http://glutenfreetravelsite.com/restaurants/

Gluten free dining and travel reviews

http://justfood.org/

Network of community food projects in New York City

http://thrv.me/7xL45S

Thrive Market. Organic and healthier non-perishable food and household items (Link is a referral. Get 25% off already discounted prices & free shipping with $49 order as of time of publication.)

http://www.celiactravel.com/cards/

Travel card for food/restaurant/gluten free communication needs when traveling to a foreign country

http://www.localharvest.org

Geographically set up to provide guides to family farms, CSAs, farmer's market, farm stands and u-pic produce for your area

https://www.ewg.org/

THE EWG'S 2017 GUIDE TO PESTICIDES IN SHOPPER'S PRODUCE ™

https://www.nal.usda.gov/afsic

USDA site with information about sustainable farming practices

https://www.nutritionaltherapy.com

Foundational Holistic Nutrition Education

https://organic.ams.usda.gov/Integrity/

A complete list of USDA-Accredited Certifying Agents

https://price-pottenger.org/

Healthy living with traditional food

https://www.TamJohn.com

DIY Wellness ™ Tips & Recipes

Personalized Wellness Coaching

Corporate & Community Wellness Presentations/Training

https://www.verywell.com/dining out gluten-free-start here 563079

Tips to dine out gluten free

https://www.westonaprice.org/

Information on nutrition and health via traditional foodways

References

Brogan, K. (2016). *A Mind of Your Own: The Truth About Depression and How Women Can Heal Their Bodies to Reclaim Their Lives.* New York: Harper Wave.

Douillard, J. (2017). *Eat Wheat: Scientific AND Clinically-Proven Approach TO Safely Bringing Wheat AND Dairy Back INTO Your Diet.* New York: Morgan James Publishing.

Douillard, J. (2000). *The 3-Season Diet: Eat the Way Nature Intended: Lost Weight, Beat Food Cravings, Get Fit.* New York: Three Rivers Press.

Emmerich, M. (2017). Keto Restaurant Favorites: *More than 175 Tasty Classic Recipes Made Fast, Fresh, and Healthy.* Las Vegas: Victory Belt Publishing Inc.

Fallon, S. & Enig, M. (1999*). Nourishing Traditions: The Cookbook that Challenges Politically Correct Nutrition and the Diet Dictocrats.* Brandywine: NewTrends Publishing, Inc.

Green, P.H.R., & Jones, R. (2016). *Gluten Exposed: The Science Behind the Hype and How to Navigate to a Healthy, Symptom-Free Life.* New York: HarperCollins.

Hay, L., Khadro, A., Dane, H., (2014). *Loving Yourself to Great Health: Thoughts & Food – the Ultimate Diet.* Carlsbad: Hay House, Inc.

Helfer, M. E., Kempe, R. S., & Krugman, R. D. (1997). *The Battered Child* (5th ed.). Chicago, IL: University of Chicago Press.

http://acestudy.org/the-ace-score.html

http://americanradioworks.publicradio.org/features/gmos_india/history.html

http://autoimmune.pathology.jhmi.edu/faqs.cfm

http://blogs.usda.gov/2013/05/17/organic-101-can-gmos-be-used-in-organic-products/

http://foodfacts.mercola.com/sprouts.html

http://fortune.com/2016/07/31/gmo-labeling-bill/

http://hrat.yale.edu/elic/summaries/hunter-gatherers

http://landofpuregold.com/the-pdfs/Excitotoxins.pdf

http://livinghistoryfarm.org/farmxinginthe40s/pests_01.html

http://onlinelibrary.wiley.com/doi/10.1046/j.1365-2796.1996.41875000.x/full)

http://soilandhealth.org/wp-content/uploads/02/0201hyglibcat/020108.coca.pdf

http://wholegrainscouncil.org/whole-grain-stamp

http://www.alternet.org/food/9-shocking-facts-you-need-know-about-sugar

https://www.cdc.gov/obesity/data/adult.html

https://www.consumerreports.org/cro/2014/10/where-gmos-hide-in-your-food/index.htm

http://www.consumerreports.org/cro/magazine/2015/01/how-much-arsenic-is-in-your-rice/index.htm

http://www.csaceliacs.org/history_of_celiac_disease.jsp

http://www.dadamo.com/B2blogs/blogs/index.php/2004/02/07/cyanocobalamin-versus-methylcobalamin?blog=27

http://www.fda.gov/Food/GuidanceRegulation/GuidanceDocumentsRegulatoryInformation/LabelingNutrition/ucm456090.htm

http://www.fda.gov/NewsEvents/Newsroom/PressAnnouncements/ucm363474.htm

http://www.health.harvard.edu/blog/eating-too-much-added-sugar-increases-the-risk-of-dying-with-heart-disease-201402067021)

http://www.health.state.mn.us/divs/hpcd/chp/cdrr/nutrition/facts/wholegrains.html

http://www.heart.org/HEARTORG/HealthyLiving/HealthyEating/HealthyDietGoals/Sugars-and-Carbohydrates_UCM_303296_Article.jsp#.WMM_6qPrvIU

http://www.jmsmucker.com/smuckers-corporate/smuckers-history

http://www.kellogghistory.com/history.html

http://www.mayoclinic.org/diseases-conditions/celiac-disease/symptoms-causes/dxc-20214627

http://www.mayoclinic.org/diseases-conditions/heart-disease/expert-answers/grass-fed-beef/FAQ-20058059

http://www.mindbodygreen.com/0-28707/could-going-gluten-free-cause-inflammation-a-doctor-explains.html?utm_source=mbg&utm_medium=email&utm_content=daily&utm_campaign=170228

http://www.naturalnews.com/034899_proteolytic_enzymes_metabolism_digestion.html

http://www.nutrition.org/fiber

http://www.nutritionfacts.org/fiber

http://www.uchospitals.edu/pdf/uch_007937.pdf

https://celiac.org/live-gluten-free/glutenfreediet/what-is-gluten/

https://celiac.org/live-gluten-free/glutenfreediet/sources-of-gluten/#O823Tu1EBeHUHJgG.99

https://chriskresser.com/harmful-or-harmless-guar-gum-locust-bean-gum-and-more/

https://chriskresser.com/harmful-or-harmless-xanthan-gum/

https://genographic.nationalgeographic.com/development-of-agriculture/

https://ghr.nlm.nih.gov/gene/HLA-B

https://nutritionfacts.org/2013/05/02/are-microgreens-healthier/

https://organic.ams.usda.gov/Integrity/

https://training.seer.cancer.gov/anatomy/lymphatic/

https://vsearch.nlm.nih.gov/vivisimo/cgi-bin/query-meta?v%3Aproject=medlineplus&v%3Asources=medlineplus-bundle&query=celiac+disease&_ga=1.243545543.331371724.1487373416

https://www.aaaai.org/Aaaai/media/MediaLibrary/PDF%20Documents/Libraries/EL-food-allergies-vs-intolerance-patient.pdf

https://www.ams.usda.gov/rules-regulations/organic/labeling

https://www.cdc.gov/diabetes/statistics/prev/national/figbyage.htm

https://www.cdc.gov/obesity/data/adult.html

https://www.choosemyplate.gov/

https://www.cnpp.usda.gov/sites/default/files/archived_projects/MiniPoster.pdf

https://www.consumerreports.org/food-safety/gras-hidden-ingredients-in-your-food/

https://www.consumerreports.org/cro/2014/10/where-gmos-hide-in-your-food/index.htm

https://www.fda.gov/Food/IngredientsPackagingLabeling/GRAS/

https://www.fda.gov/Food/IngredientsPackagingLabeling/GRAS/SCOGS/ucm261246.htm

https://www.hsph.harvard.edu/nutritionsource/carbohydrates/fiber/

https://www.hsph.harvard.edu/nutritionsource/whole-grains/

https://www.khanacademy.org/test-prep/nclex-rn/gastrointestinal-diseases/celiac-disease-rn/a/what-is-celiac-disease

https://www.merriam-webster.com/dictionary/food

https://www.ncbi.nlm.nih.gov/pmc/articles/PMC3900881/

https://www.ncbi.nlm.nih.gov/books/NBK26871/

https://www.nongmoproject.org/product-verification/

https://www.oncologynutrition.org/erfc/healthy-nutrition-now/sugar-and-cancer/

https://www.thoughtco.com/history-of-the-can-and-can-opener-1991487

https://www.webmd.com/food-recipes/features/sugar-shockers-foods-surprisingly-high-in-sugar

Hyman, M. (2016). Eat Fat, *Get Thin: Why the Fat We Eat Is the Key to Sustained Weight Loss and Vibrant Health.* New York: Little, Brown and Company.

Lau, N. G. (2013, June). Markers of Celiac Disease and Gluten Sensitivity in Children with Autism. *PLoS ONE, 8*(6), 1-6. doi:10.1371/journal.pone.0066155

Marieb, E. & Hoehn K. (2013). *Human Anatomy & Physiology: Ninth Edition.* Glenview: Pearson Education, Inc.

Murray, J.A. (2014). Going Gluten Free: *ESSENTIAL GUIDE to Managing Celiac Disease and Related Conditions.* New York: Time Home Entertainment Inc.

Northrup, C. (2012). The *Wisdom of Menopause: Creating Physical and Emotional Health During the Change.* Random House: New York.

Pollan, M. (2008). *In Defense of Food: An Eater's Manifesto.* New York: Penguin Group.

Price, W. (2014). Nutrition and Physical Degeneration (6th ed.). Lemon Grove, CA: Price-Pottenger Nutrition Foundation.

Samuel, A., & Seneff, S. (2013). *Glyphosate, pathways to modern diseases II: Celiac sprue and gluten intolerance. Journal of Interdisciplinary Toxicology, Vol. 6(4): 159-184. doi:10.2478/-intox-2013-0026*

Yang, Q., Zhang, Z., Gregg, E., Flanders, W.D., Merritt, R., & Hu, F. (2014). Added Sugar Intake and Cardiovascular Diseases Mortality Among US Adults. *The Journal of the American Medical Association Internal Medicine, 174(4):516-524.* doi:10.1001/jamainter-med.2013.13563

Made in the USA
Columbia, SC
15 February 2018